# The NATURAL SKIN CARE RECIPE BOOK

Get that Glowing Look with Homemade Beauty Products
Made from Non-Toxic, Eco-Friendly Ingredients

## KATE JONES

Creator of My Plastic Free Home and Owner of The Natural Living Shop

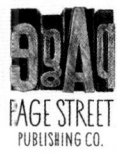

PAGE STREET
PUBLISHING CO.

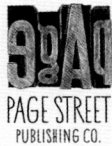

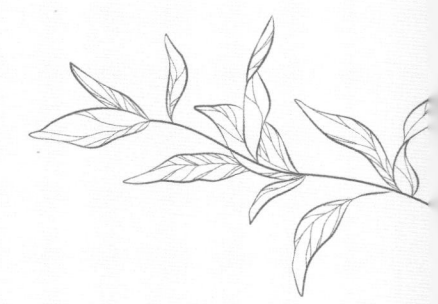

Copyright © 2024 Kate Jones

First published in 2024 by
Page Street Publishing Co.
27 Congress Street, Suite 1511
Salem, MA 01970
www.pagestreetpublishing.com

All rights reserved. No part of this book may be reproduced or used, in any form or by any means, electronic or mechanical, without prior permission in writing from the publisher.

Distributed by Macmillan, sales in Canada by The Canadian Manda Group.

28  27  26  25  24      1  2  3  4  5

ISBN-13: 979-8-89003-065-8

Library of Congress Control Number: 2023945218

Edited by Franny Donington-Ayad
Cover and book design by Meg Baskis for Page Street Publishing Co.
Photography by Alejandra Sinclair

Printed and bound in the United States of America

Page Street Publishing protects our planet by donating to nonprofits like The Trustees, which focuses on local land conservation.

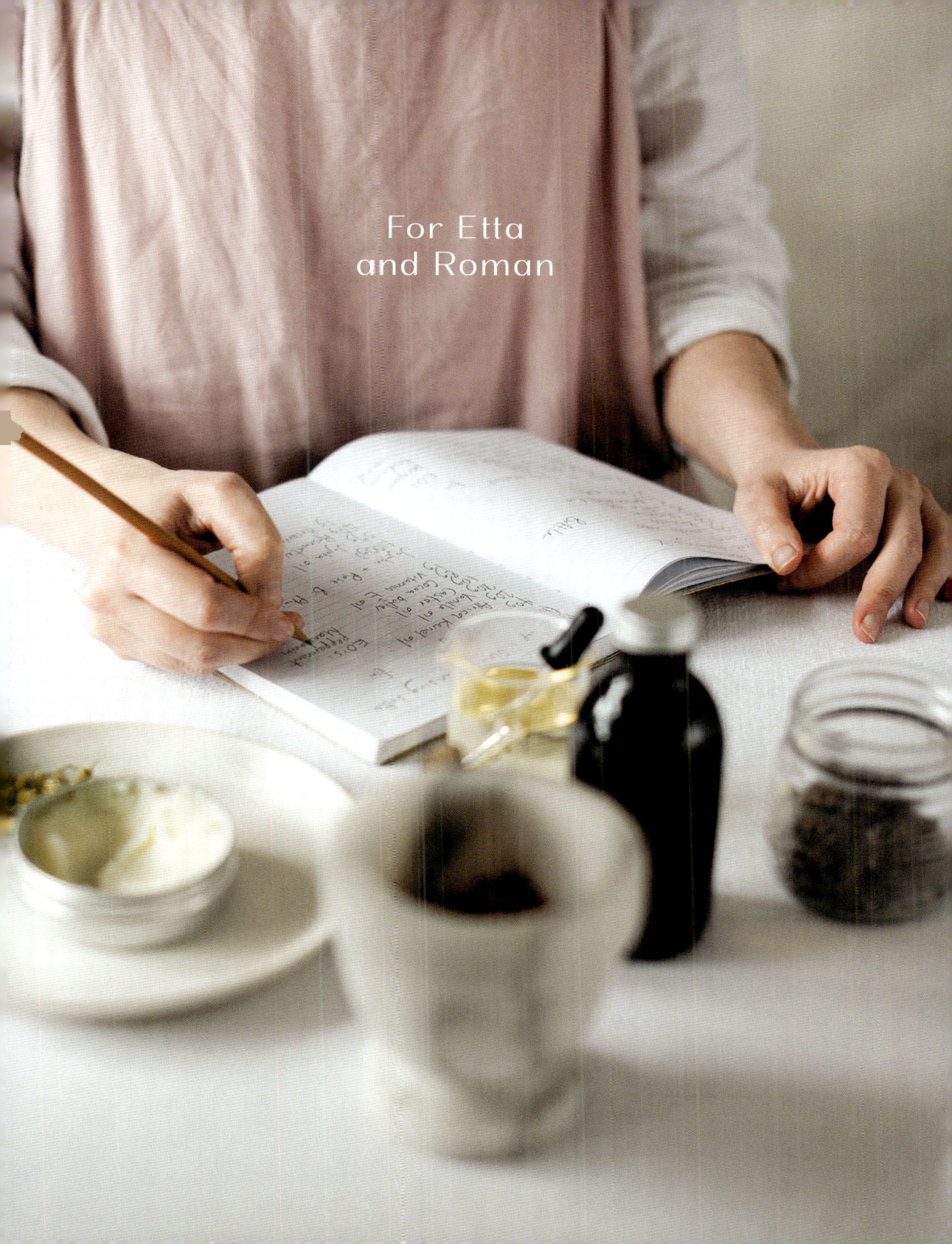

For Etta and Roman

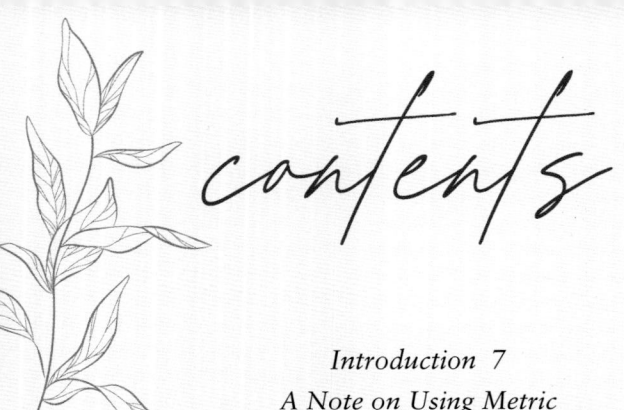

# contents

*Introduction* 7
*A Note on Using Metric Measurements* 9
*Take Precaution: Test Your Products* 9

## CLEANSERS AND TONERS • 11
Get the Glow Cleansing Butter  13
Relax and Restore Creamy Cleanser  14
Nourishing Jojoba and Rose Bi-Phase Cleanser  17
Botanical Micellar Cleansing Milk  18
Relaxing Lavender Toner and Face Spritz  21
Hydrating Rose Water Toning Bar  22
Calm and Tone Chamomile Sphere  25

## FACE OILS, LOTIONS AND BALMS • 27
Glow Face Oil  29
Relax and Restore Facial Oil  30
Nourishing Jojoba Face Lotion  33
Protective Balm  34

## BODY LOTIONS AND BUTTERS • 37
Nourishing Vitamin E Body Lotion  39
Calming Whipped Body Butter  40
Buttery Body Lotion  43
Indulgent Whipped Body Butter  44

## LOTION BARS • 47
Deep Muscle Massaging Bar  49
Relaxing Massage Lotion Bar  50
Everyday Rituals Massaging Lotion Bar  53

## BALMS • 55
After-Sun Soothing Balm  57
Botanical Bruise Balm  58
Hydrating Lip Balm  61
Repairing Lip Balm  62
Aromatherapy Massage Lotion Balm  65

## SCRUBS • 67
Indulgent Sugar Body Scrub  69
Glowing Face Polish  70
Plumping Peppermint and Vanilla Lip Scrub  73

## FACE MASKS • 75
Rose Clay Hydrating Face Mask  77
Green Clay Deep Cleanse Face Mask  78
Kaolin Caring Clay Mask  81
Calming Oat Face Mask  82

## TREATMENT OILS • 85
Hair Growth Oil  87
Soothe Your Skin Massage Oil  88
Eyebrow Growth Oil  91
Nourishing Cuticle Balm  92

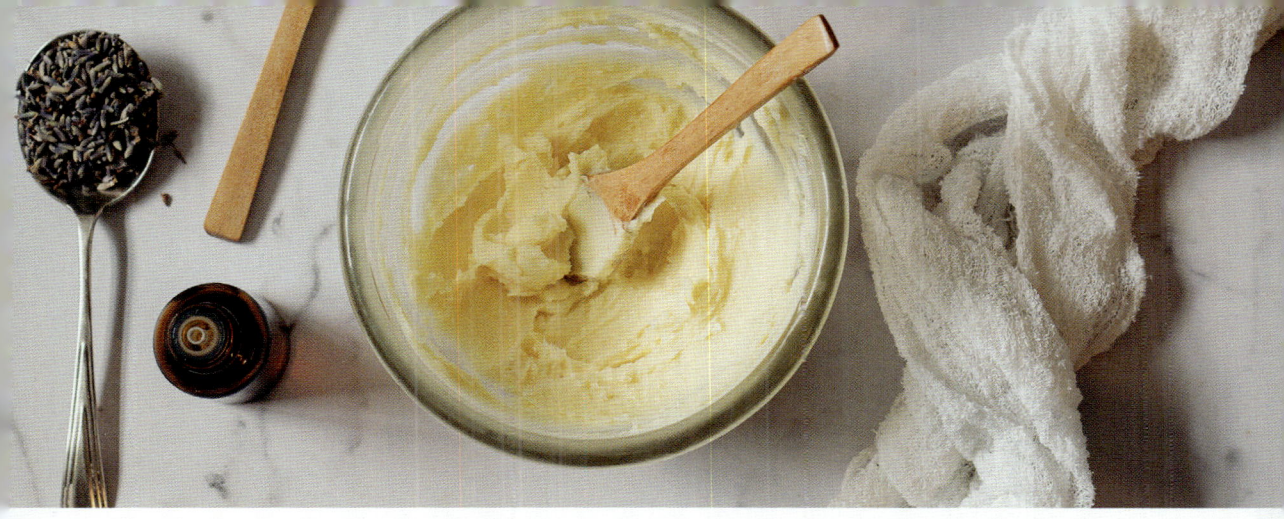

## BATH INDULGENCE · 95
Calming Bath Melts  97
Uplifting Bath Melts  98
Relax and Unwind Bath Bombs  101
Lovely Bubbles Bath Bombs  102
Soothing Bath and Body Oil  105
Botanical Bath and Body Oil  106
Herbal Infused Bath Salts  109
Floral Bath Salts  110
Wake Up Shower Steamers  113
Sleepy Time Shower Steamers  114

## BOTANICAL OILS · 117
Lavender Infused Oil  119
Calendula Infused Oil  120
Rosemary Infused Oil  123
Rose Petal Infused Oil  124
Chamomile Flower Infused Oil  127
Rosehip Infused Oil  128
Vanilla Pod Infused Oil  131

## BOTANICAL HYDROSOLS · 133
DIY Rose Water Hydrosol  135
DIY Chamomile Hydrosol  136
DIY Lavender Hydrosol  139
DIY Rosemary Hydrosol  140
DIY Witch Hazel Hydrosol  143

## METHODS AND GUIDES · 145
The Double Boiler Method  146
Finding a Trace Line  146
Troubleshooting Butters and Balms  147
A Guide to Making Infused Oils  148
A Guide to Sterilizing Jars  149
A Guide to Preservatives  149
Essential Oil Information  150
Equipment List  151
Ingredients List  151
Shelf Stability of Ingredients  152

*About the Author  153*
*Acknowledgments  154*
*Make Your Own Recipe!  155*
*Index  156*

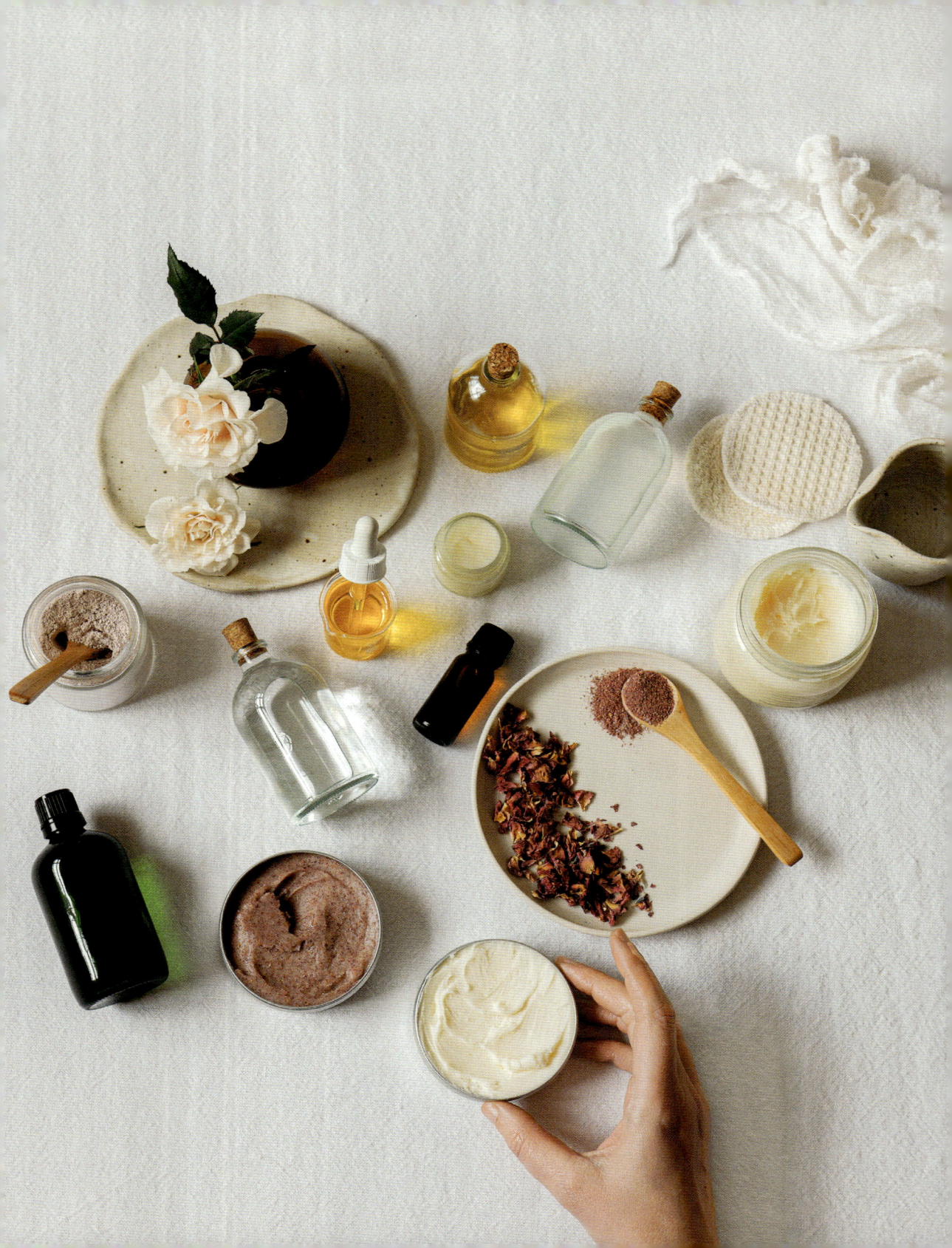

# INTRODUCTION

Welcome to *The Natural Skin Care Recipe Book*. This book is packed full of simple recipes that you can make on your kitchen table that feed your skin with beautiful botanicals, rich butters and hydrating oils.

Not only is this collection of recipes good for you, but it is good for the planet too. I have focused on a selection of raw ingredients that are organically sourced, palm oil free and abundant in nature. I am going to show you all of the different ways that you can use these ingredients to make an array of different skin care products so that you can simplify your skin care routine and feel confident in the choices that you are making for your skin.

I have chosen to focus on a range of raw ingredients that can be used interchangeably throughout the book. I remember that the first time I attempted to create my own skin care products I became quickly overwhelmed with how many different ingredients I needed to source, and I found it really difficult to make a skin care routine without feeling that I was being quite wasteful by just experimenting! Thankfully, I have tested and perfected my recipes so that you can dive in successfully.

It really is empowering when you learn how many different ways a single ingredient can be used to make oils, lotions, butters, balms, scrubs and so much more! I have selected a number of recipes for each skin care step so that you can find exactly what you feel works best for your skin type. Along the way, I will also be explaining why I chose certain ingredients and factors to be aware of when using the ingredients so that you can develop your understanding of what works and gain confidence in making your own skin care products. A full list of ingredients used in this book is also available on page 151 to make it easy for you to get started.

With the power of natural ingredients that are good for you and for our planet, we can hydrate, soothe, cleanse and nourish our skin for a glowing look and healthy feel.

I can't wait to begin this journey with you.

Kate x

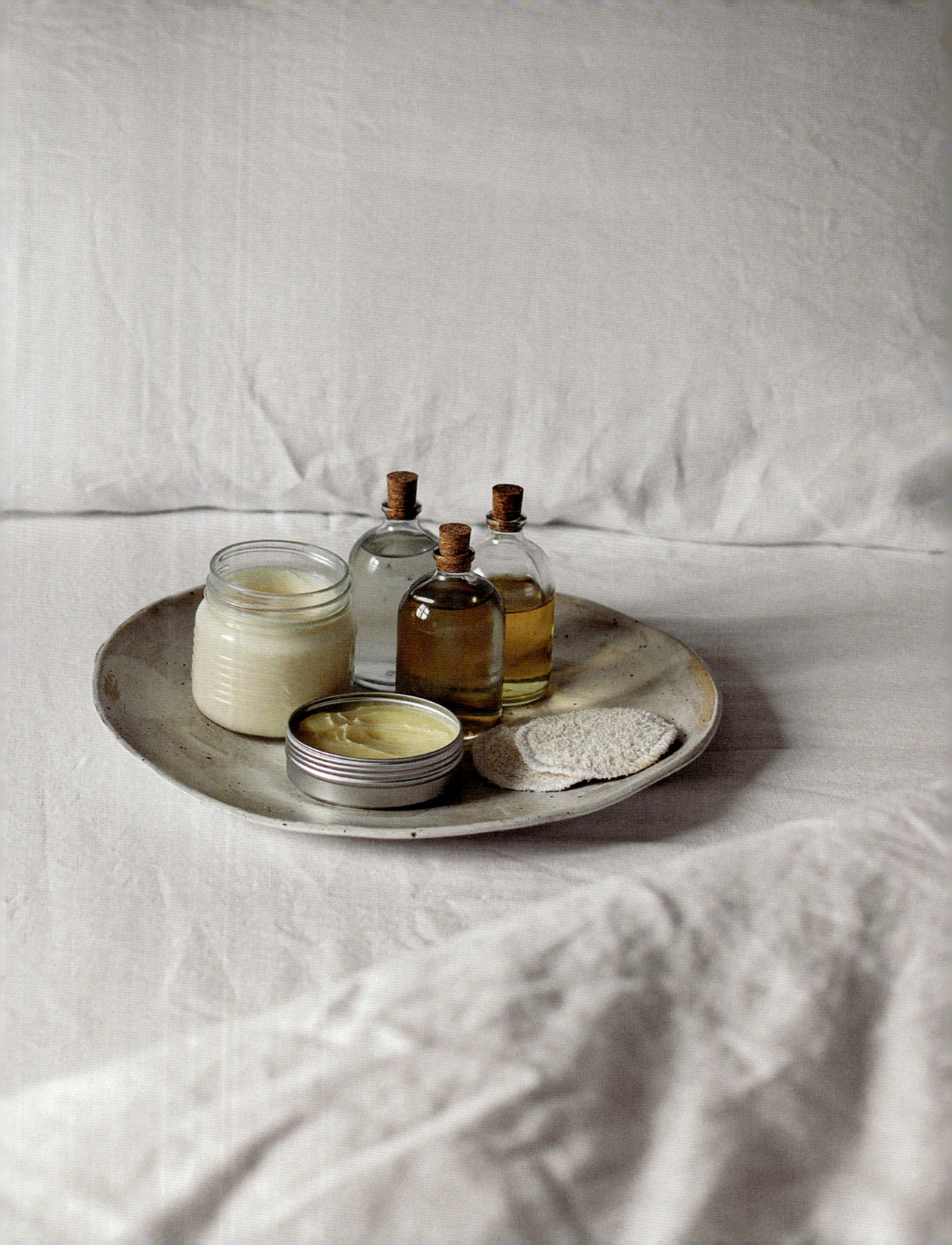

# A NOTE ON USING METRIC MEASUREMENTS

Throughout this guide, I will be discussing specific measurements for each recipe. There are a number of recipes that need exact measurements to make safe and effective skin care products that are shelf-stable and not irritating when applied to your skin. For that reason, throughout this guide, I have provided metric measurements such as grams and milliliters. I strongly recommend using those rather than volume measurements, such as tablespoons and cups, to be as accurate as possible. I always recommend using a 0.01-gram jewelry scale for this reason (equipment recommendations are discussed further on page 151).

When it comes to adding powerful ingredients like essential oils, which you need to use very sparsely to be safe, it's important to measure small amounts, which a jewelry scale is perfect for. The same goes for the preservatives we will add into some of our products, which we need to be very exact with.

# TAKE PRECAUTION: TEST YOUR PRODUCTS

Before using any new skin care product, I strongly recommend conducting a patch test to ensure compatibility with your skin.

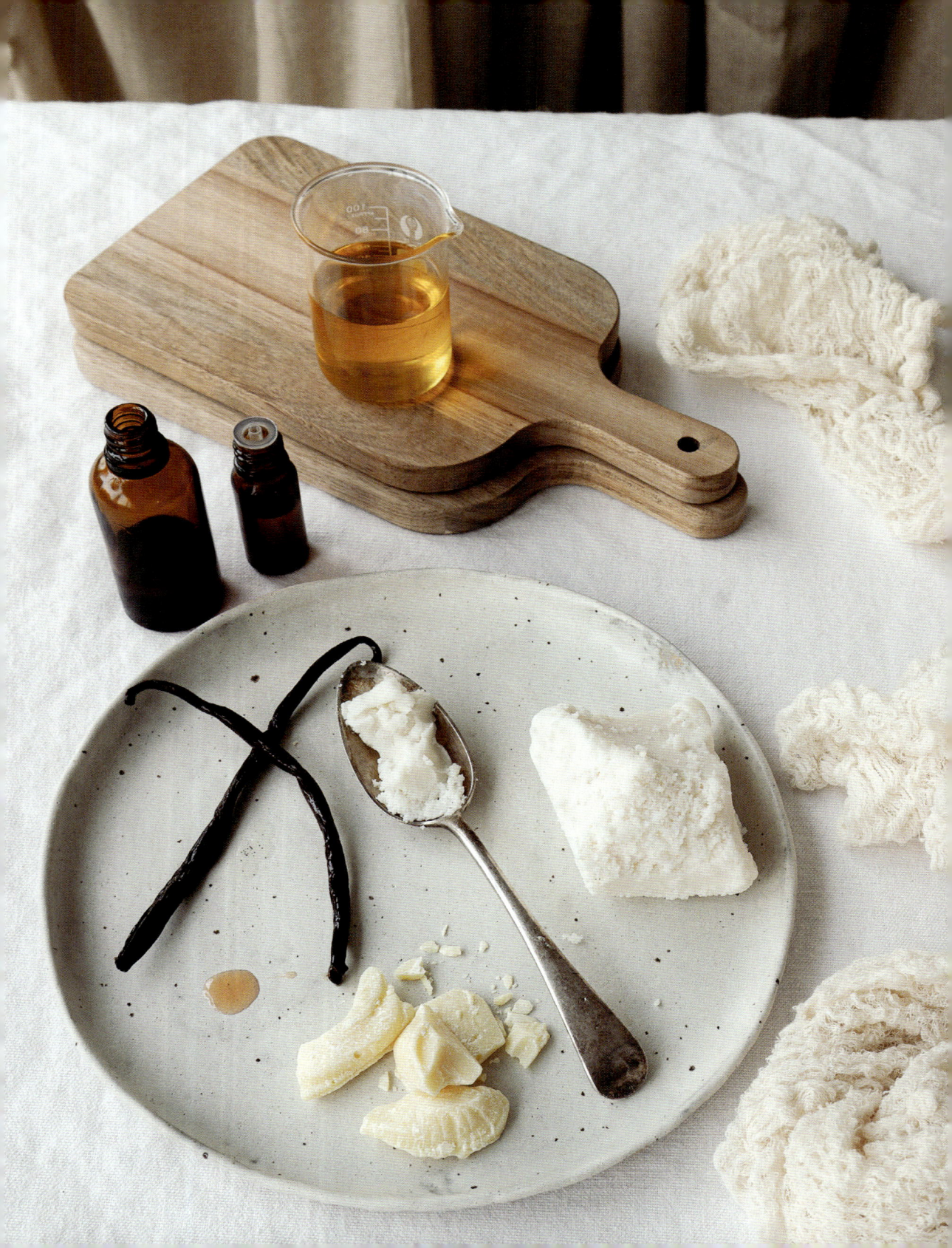

# CLEANSERS AND TONERS

I will begin our skin care guide with four types of cleansers that you can create to rid your skin of the day's grime and relax into your skin care routine. For me, cleansers are one of the most important steps in your skin care routine. They help you begin your day refreshed and revitalized in the mornings, and they also help you to end your day in the perfect way by ridding your skin of makeup, pollution and even stress to reset your day and settle into a lovely nighttime routine. Cleansers are the first step in your skin care routine, and you can use them on their own or as part of a double cleanse if you feel that your skin really needs some attention. Follow up with a toner and your skin will be perfectly prepped.

Toners are a very simple part of your skin care routine and help remove any last trace of grime or impurities stuck in your pores after cleansing. They also help to restore your skin's natural pH balance and prepare your skin to better absorb moisture. I have included two different ways I love to make toners. One is a liquid toner that I like to add to a spray bottle and spritz my face with. The second way I love to make toners is by freezing them into bars and storing them in the freezer. This is a beautiful way to use your toner, refresh your skin and reduce puffiness too!

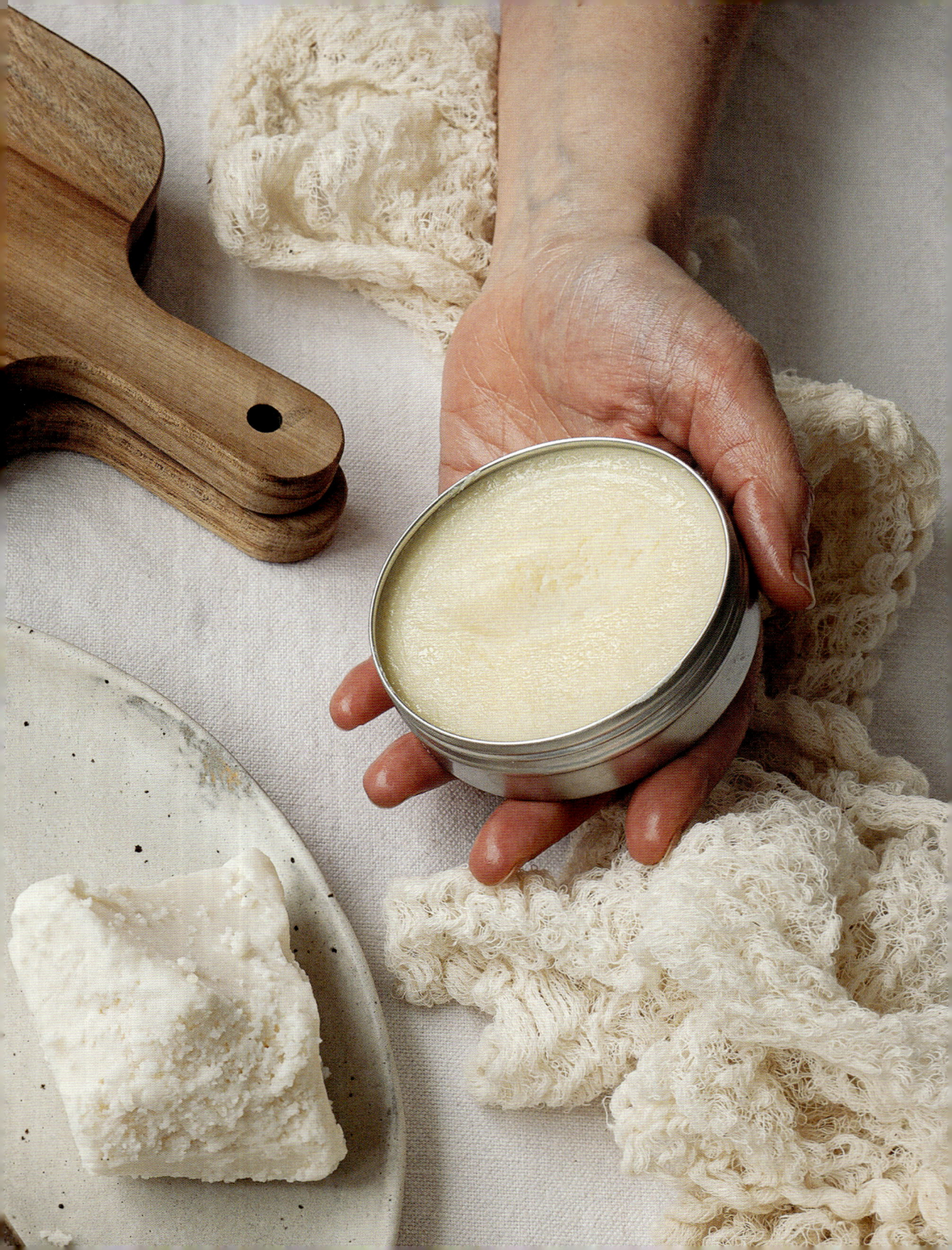

# GET THE GLOW CLEANSING BUTTER

*This creamy cleanser is so nourishing and the perfect consistency to massage deeply into the skin and prepare you for the day. It is rich in vitamin A, which plays a crucial role in skin health and helps to promote skin regeneration and maintain a healthy complexion. I like to sit down and massage this cleanser into my skin, allowing the butters and oils to nourish and the essential oils to invigorate my skin. Gently remove this cleanser with a warm muslin cloth for the most nourished, rejuvenated skin.*

*Makes* 1 medium-sized tin (100 g [½ cup])

40 g (2½ tbsp) mango butter

20 g (1½ tbsp) apricot kernel oil

20 g (1½ tbsp) Vanilla Pod Infused Oil (page 131)

10 g (3 tsp) castor oil

8 g (3 tsp) cocoa butter

0.5 g mandarin essential oil

1 g vitamin E oil

0.2 g peppermint essential oil

Using the double boiler method, gently melt the mango butter, apricot kernel oil, Vanilla Pod Infused Oil, castor oil and cocoa butter until it is a liquid consistency. You can make your own double boiler by placing a bowl over a pot of simmering water. Keep the water simmering but not boiling, and make sure the bowl doesn't touch the water. Melt the butter until it is liquid (see page 146 for more detailed information about the double boiler method).

Place your mixture in the fridge. When the mixture has cooled to below 77°F (25°C), add the mandarin essential oil, vitamin E oil and peppermint essential oil. This should take 10 to 15 minutes to cool. Stir to combine all of the ingredients. I like to use a small whisk for this.

Add to a clean, sterile container and place in the refrigerator to cool. Take it out and stir occasionally while it cools, until you see a trace line in the cleanser, and allow to set for 24 hours. See page 146 for more information on trace lines.

To use, take a small amount (about the size of a blueberry) and massage into the skin for a couple of minutes.

Remove with a dampened muslin cloth or face towel.

## Get to Know Your Ingredients!

This is a soft cleanser that will change from solid to liquid as you use it and get to work quickly on your skin. I have used castor oil in this recipe, which is a very thick oil and has a slow absorption rate. This makes it a great addition to your cream-based cleanser and helps to draw out all of the day's grime like a magnet. I adore adding peppermint essential oil to my cleanser, as I find that it helps to cool my skin and wake me up in the morning.

# RELAX AND RESTORE CREAMY CLEANSER

*This is a deeply luxurious and relaxing cleansing balm. I feel that cleansers are the most underrated product, as they prepare your skin for the day and also prepare your skin for the night. This creamy cleanser contains oils that are slower to penetrate, and I like to take the time to massage them into my skin as part of my nighttime routine. The ingredients used in this recipe are rich in antioxidants and help fight free radicals. Free radicals can cause damage to cells and proteins, contributing to aging. Antioxidants like vitamin E help combat free radicals by stabilizing them, reducing their potential harm and supporting overall health. The botanical infused oils and essential oils I have chosen for this recipe also help to prepare me for a restful night's sleep.*

*Makes* 1 medium-sized tin (100 g [½ cup])

24 g (1½ tbsp) cocoa butter

24 g (1½ tbsp) mango butter

20 g (1½ tbsp) sweet almond oil

20 g (1½ tbsp) Lavender Infused Oil (page 119)

10 g (3 tsp) castor oil

1 g vitamin E oil

0.3 g bergamot essential oil

0.2 g rosemary essential oil

0.2 g lavender essential oil

Using the double boiler method, warm the blend of the cocoa butter, mango butter, sweet almond oil, Lavender Infused Oil and castor oil until it has melted into liquid. Read more about the double boiler method on page 146.

Place your mixture in the fridge. When it has cooled to below 77°F (25°C), add the vitamin E oil, bergamot essential oil, rosemary essential oil and lavender essential oil. This should take 10 to 15 minutes to cool. Gently whisk to combine all of the ingredients.

Add to a clean, sterile container and place in the refrigerator to cool. Take it out and stir occasionally while it cools, until you see a trace line in the cleanser, and allow to set for 24 hours. See page 146 for more information on trace lines.

To use this cleanser, take a small amount (about the size of a blueberry) and rub it between the palms of your hands. Make a cup shape with your hands, bring it to your nose and deeply inhale the aroma of the essential oils to help you relax and unwind. Take the time to massage the formula into your skin, capturing all of the day's grime.

Remove with a dampened muslin cloth or face towel.

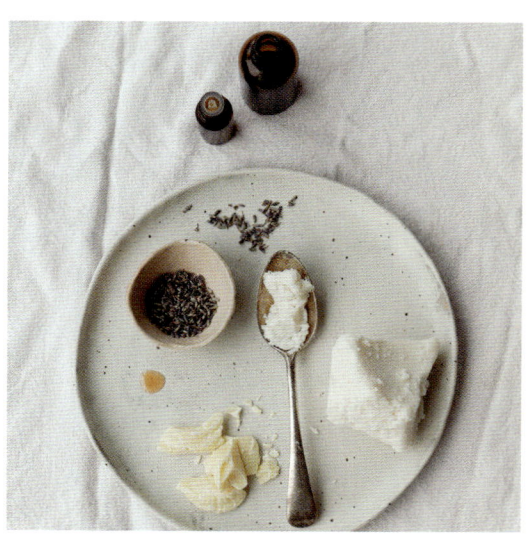

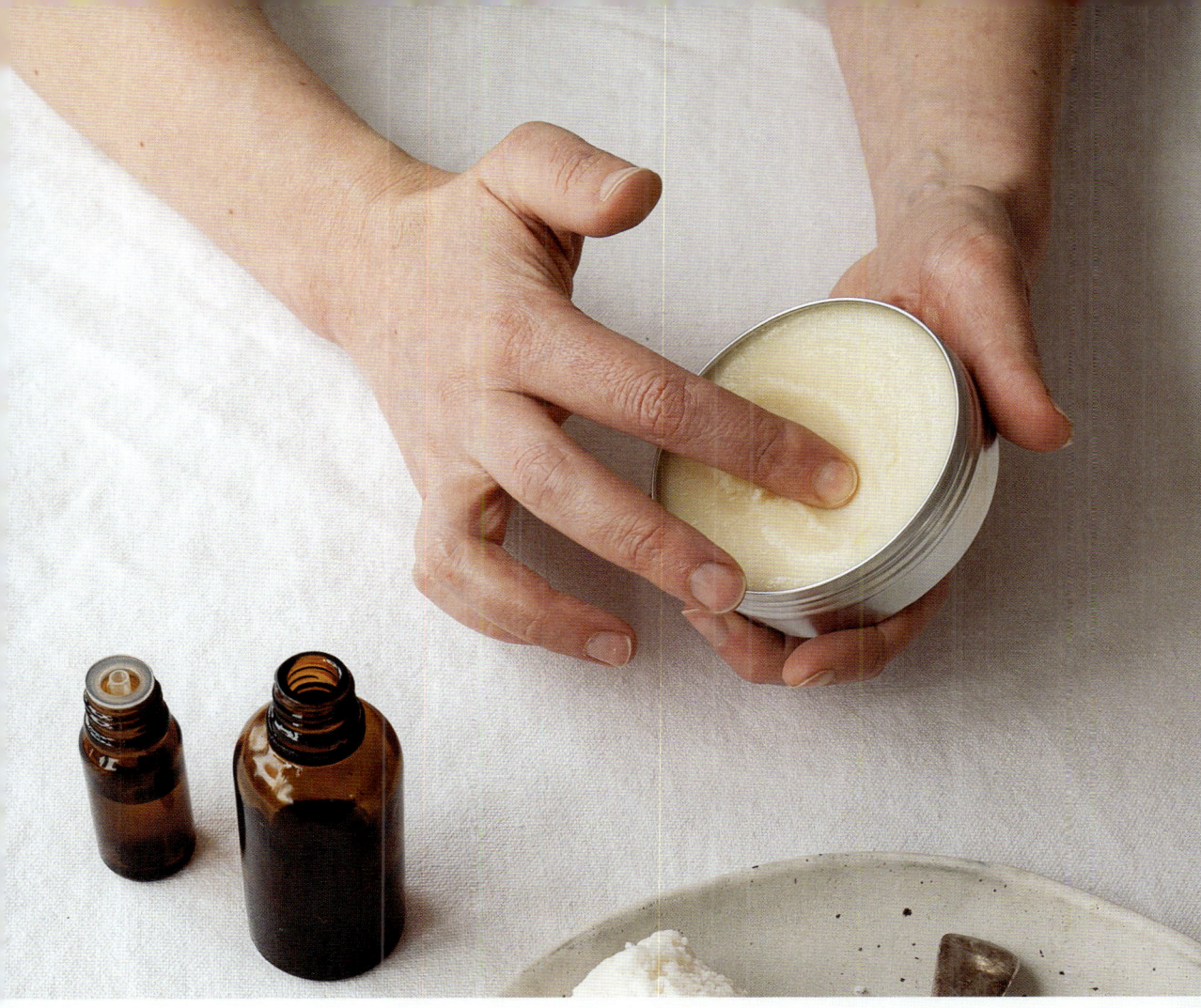

## Get to Know Your Ingredients!

Sweet almond oil is a favorite of mine to use as it's so moisturizing and hydrating, while the Lavender Infused Oil helps to soothe your skin while also promoting relaxation and reducing stress. The blend of essential oils that I have included in this recipe is also stress reducing and a great way to help you relax while you're completing your skin care routine after a stressful day!

Please make sure you adhere to the exact measurements for the essential oils. Although one or two drops of each oil may not seem like much, they are so very concentrated and contain a plentiful amount of the botanical. I discuss essential oils in more detail on page 150.

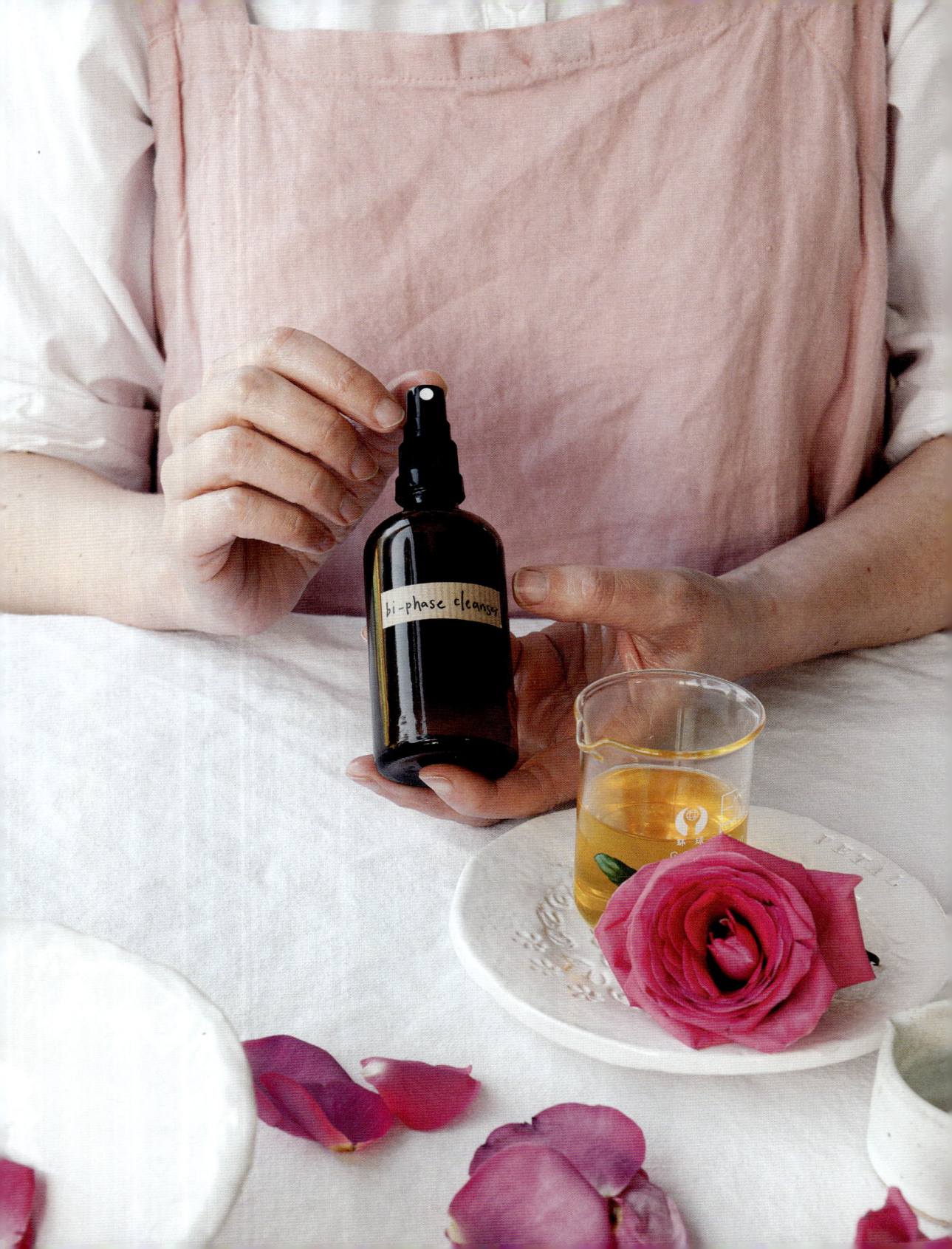

# NOURISHING JOJOBA AND ROSE BI-PHASE CLEANSER

*This is the most refreshing cleanser and so efficient at removing your makeup—you'll be astonished at how well it removes eye makeup, leaving no trace behind! This cleanser is rich in vitamins E and B complex, is noncomedogenic and helps to balance oil production in the skin, making it really useful for oily and acne-prone skin. As this is a bi-phase cleanser, you will need to shake the bottle before you use it as the oil will naturally sit on top of the hydrosol. When combined together, it will create a milky, nourishing cleanser that is gentle but very effective.*

*Makes* 1 medium-sized bottle (100 g [½ cup])

59 g (3½ tbsp) jojoba oil
40 g (2½ tbsp) DIY Rose Water Hydrosol (page 135)
1 g preservative eco

Mix the jojoba oil and Rose Water Hydrosol together. You will notice that the ingredients don't combine and instead the oil forms balls of liquid inside the hydrosol; this is perfectly normal.

Add the preservative eco to the mixture and stir to combine. Add your mixture to a clean, sterile spray bottle. Shake before use.

## Get to Know Your Ingredients!

I have added an eco-friendly preservative to this formulation. When introducing water to skin care products, there is a risk that bacteria will grow in the product, and the product will have a very limited shelf life of only a few days. Using a preservative in any formulation that includes water will make the product safe to use and give it a shelf life. Preservative eco needs to be 1 percent of the formulation, so this will make 100 grams (½ cup). If you are making 200 grams (1 cup), you would need to double the amount of preservative to make it safe. If using a different type of preservative, you will need to check the requirements of that specific preservative—see page 149 for more information about preservatives.

Jojoba oil has a long shelf life and is a fantastic moisturizer for the skin. It helps to control sebum production and works to gently unclog pores and remove grime from the skin, making it an excellent cleansing oil.

Rose Water Hydrosol is a soothing floral water that is great for irritated or acne-prone skin and is very gentle and rejuvenating.

# BOTANICAL MICELLAR CLEANSING MILK

*This is a very gentle and refreshing cleansing milk. You can use it alone or as part of a double cleanse method. I love to use it as the second part of a double cleanse method to make sure that every last impurity has been removed from my skin. This cleansing milk is pH-balanced and really hydrating too.*

*Makes* 1 medium bottle (200 ml [¾ cup])

110 g (6 tbsp) DIY Lavender Hydrosol (page 139)

69 g (4 tbsp) DIY Rose Water Hydrosol (page 135)

10 g (3 tsp) glycerine

8 g (3 tsp) organic Castile soap

2 g preservative eco

1 g citric acid granules

Mix the Lavender Hydrosol, Rose Water Hydrosol and glycerine together. Add the Castile soap and slowly combine.

Add the preservative eco to your mixture. This needs to be kept to the exact measurement to make sure that your cleanser is protected from bacteria and is shelf-stable.

Add the citric acid granules and stir to combine. You will notice that this addition takes your clear water and changes it to a milky color; this is why I call it a cleansing milk!

Transfer to a small sterile bottle. Use to cleanse your face in the morning and the evening. This can also be used as the second part of a double cleanse method and works well in conjunction with cream cleansers.

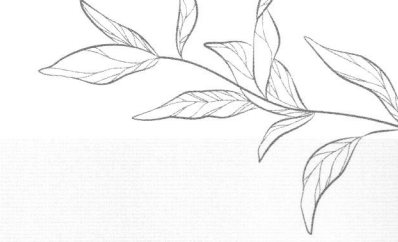

## Get to Know Your Ingredients!

Micellar waters are such a popular cleansing product because they are so gentle on the skin. I have included a small amount of surfactant in this recipe in the form of organic Castile soap. This further helps to cleanse the skin and also keeps the pH level of the micellar water at an appropriate level.

Many surfactant cleansers available to buy are actually too alkaline and, therefore, too harsh for the skin, which is why your skin can feel tight or irritated after using them. If the pH is higher than 6.5, it will need a very small amount of acidic compound to return the entire mixture to an appropriate pH level (between 4 and 6.5). I do this by adding a food-grade citric acid. As the mixture is water-based, I have added this directly. It is a very useful way of making sure your products are balanced and will not irritate your skin.

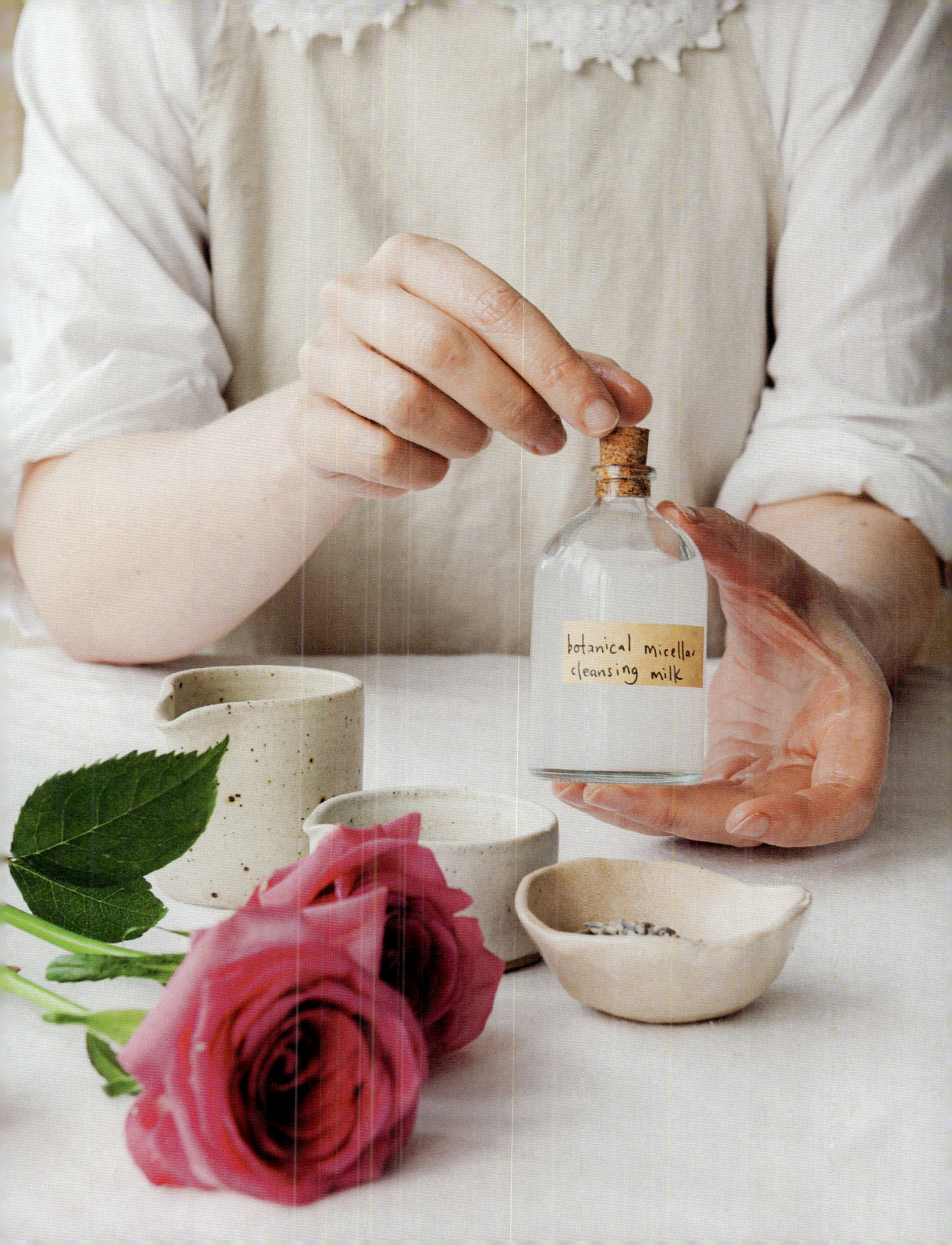

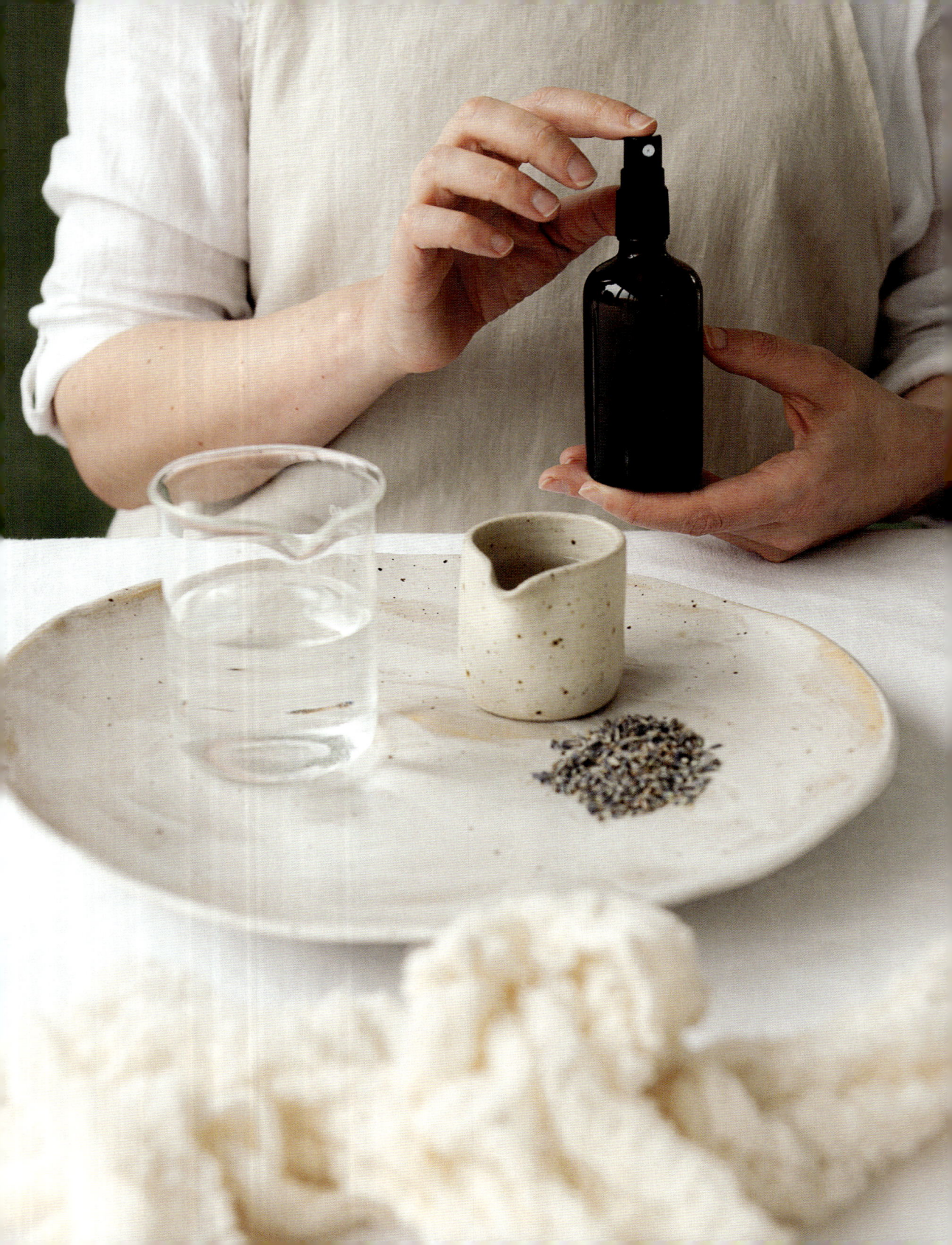

# RELAXING LAVENDER TONER AND FACE SPRITZ

*This is such a wonderful toner that is really refreshing and hydrating for your skin. The witch hazel is mildly astringent and great for oily and acne-prone skin, and the combination is anti-inflammatory too. I use it as a toner after cleansing my skin, and I also use it to refresh my skin throughout the day!*

*Makes* 1 medium-sized bottle (100 g [½ cup])

50 g (3 tbsp) DIY Lavender Hydrosol (page 139)

49 g (3 tbsp) DIY Witch Hazel Hydrosol (page 143)

1 g preservative eco

Add the Lavender Hydrosol, Witch Hazel Hydrosol and preservative eco to a bowl and stir well.

Transfer to a sterilized spray bottle for easy application—just mist your face when using!

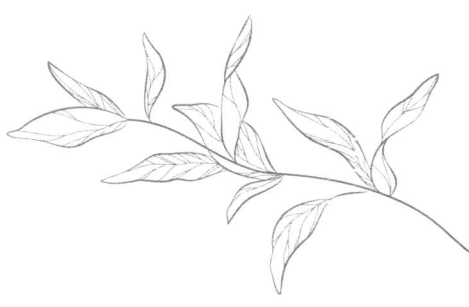

## Get to Know Your Ingredients!

Lavender Hydrosol is cooling, hydrating and toning, making it a fantastic toner to add to your beauty regimen. Witch hazel is a great ingredient for acne-prone skin and is also thought to help tone the skin and tighten pores. In addition to this, it has cooling properties and is great for sensitive skin. These two hydrosols blend perfectly to make a gentle toner. This is such a simple recipe and you can experiment with different hydrosols when making this toner. Another favorite of mine is rose water, which is also hydrating, naturally brightening and helps to improve redness in the skin.

# HYDRATING ROSE WATER TONING BAR

*I happened upon the idea of making these bars as I was looking for a DIY alternative to using a frozen face globe for my skin. I find them so useful for waking up my skin and reducing puffiness. The rose water also helps to reduce redness and irritation and is a natural way to brighten the skin.*

*Makes* 1 bar (40 g [2 oz])

40 g (2½ tbsp) DIY Rose Water Hydrosol (page 135)

Add the Rose Water Hydrosol to a silicone mold and freeze overnight.

Sweep over your skin to use as a cooling toner and return to the freezer after each use.

### Get to Know Your Ingredients!

Rose water helps to hydrate and brighten the skin and balance the skin's pH levels, making it a perfect ingredient as a toner. Freezing your toner into bar form means that you don't need to add a preservative to it. It's also a great way to use a toner as the frozen bar will refresh your skin while the rose water is also toning your skin! Please note that the addition of botanicals as used in the image is not necessary for the recipe.

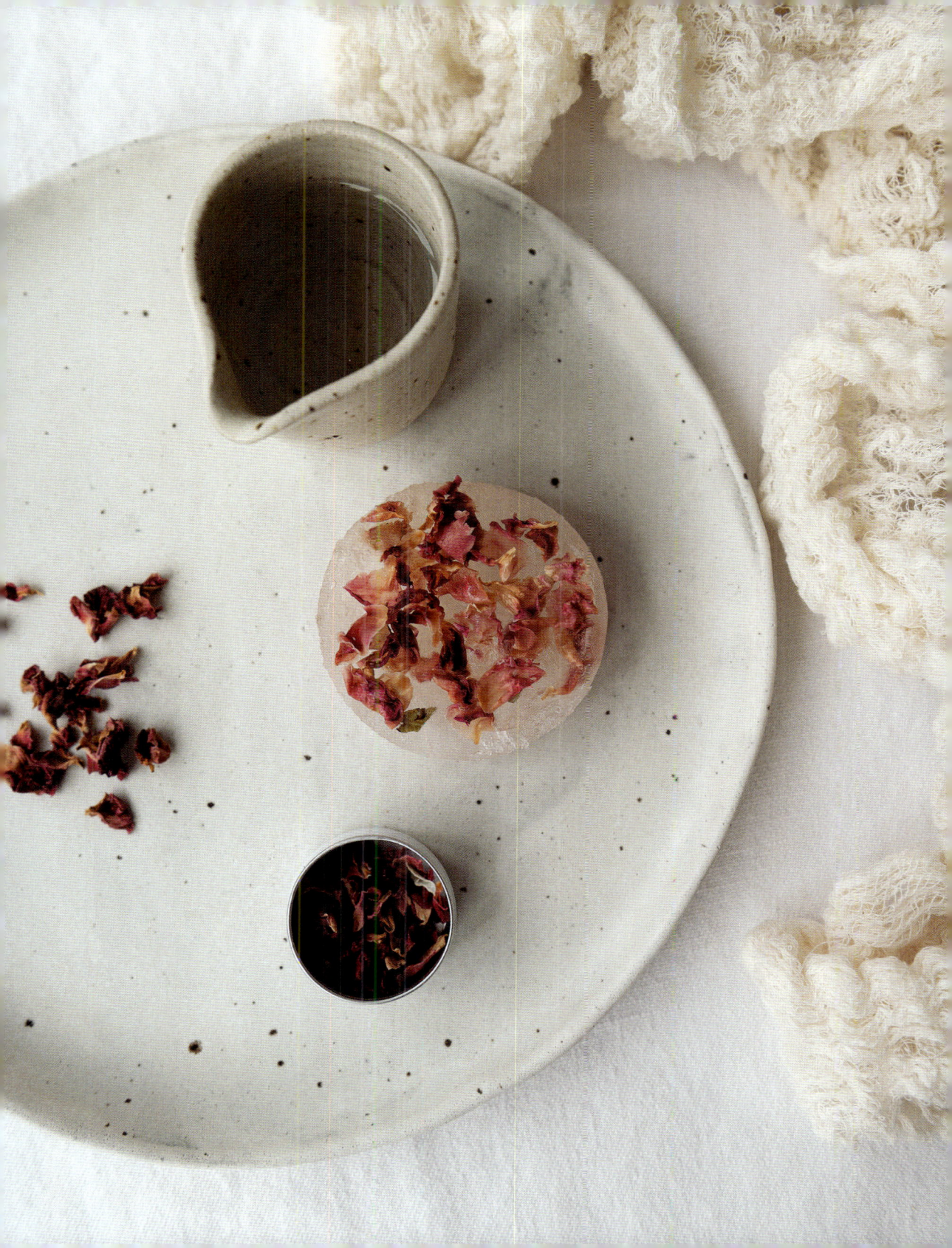

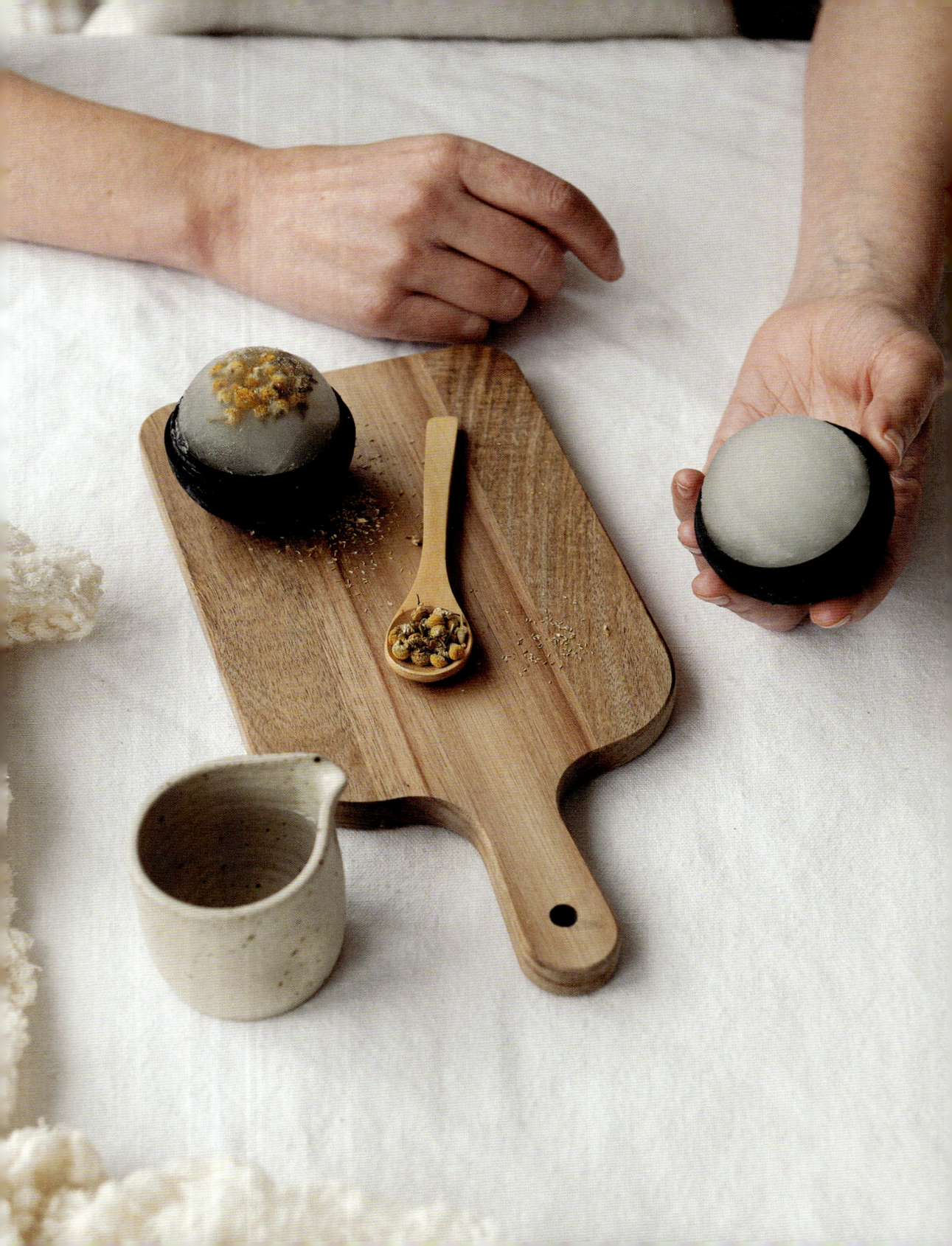

# CALM AND TONE CHAMOMILE SPHERE

*Similar to the Hydrating Rose Water Toning Bar (page 22), I enjoy freezing this toner, and this time, I have used a spherical mold. It's great for sweeping over your face in the morning and the shape helps to massage all the contours of your skin. Additionally, it is soothing and calming and helps to promote a more even skin tone.*

*Makes* 1 sphere (60 g [2.5 oz])

60 g (3½ tbsp) DIY Chamomile Hydrosol (page 136)

Add the Chamomile Hydrosol to a spherical mold and freeze overnight.

Sweep over your skin to use as a cooling toner; the curved edges of the mold will also allow you to massage your skin and relieve any puffiness.

Return to the freezer after each use.

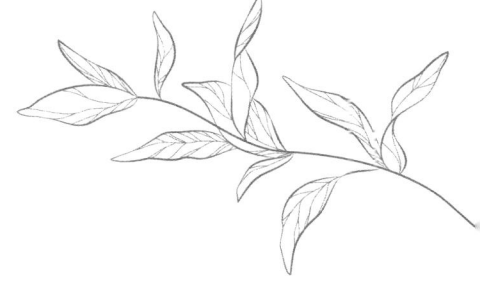

## Get to Know Your Ingredients!

Chamomile Hydrosol is so gentle and hydrating and can help soothe irritated or sensitive skin. It helps alleviate redness and puffiness and is the perfect ingredient in these frozen globes to help smooth and tone the skin. Please note that the addition of botanicals as used in the image is not necessary for the recipe.

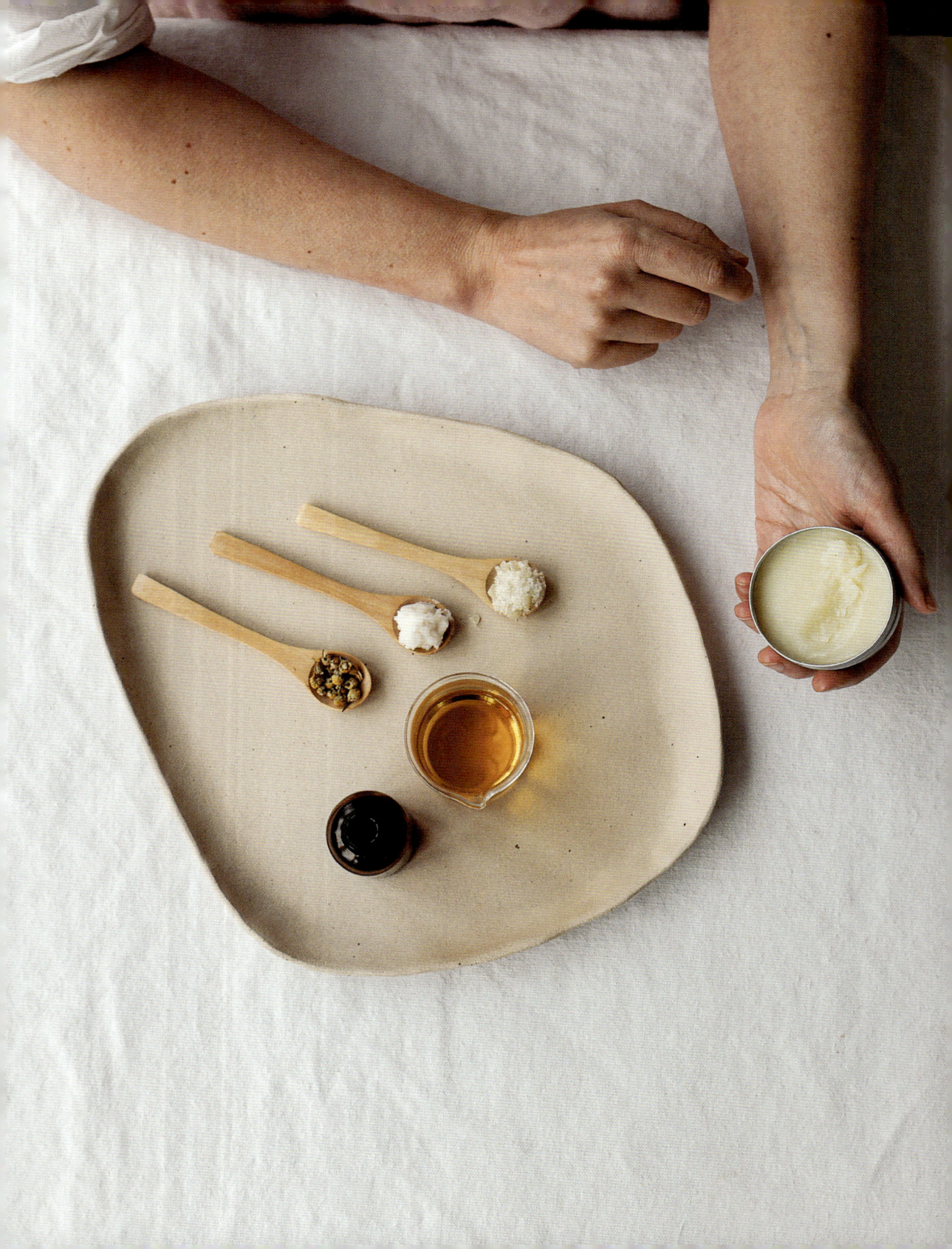

# FACE OILS, LOTIONS AND BALMS

Having oily skin myself meant that I shied away from using oils on my face until I was in my thirties, and I put that down as one of the biggest mistakes that I have made when it comes to skin care! Facial oils are great for all skin types, as they help to regulate the sebum production in your skin while keeping your skin supple and hydrated. In the winter months, I swap between using a facial oil to lotions and balms, which are rich and protect my skin from the harsh weather. The lotions and balms that I make for my skin are deeply luxurious and moisturizing and, again, don't be scared to use them on your face because they are oil-based. You will only need a pea-sized amount, and they are all made using noncomedogenic ingredients and will not clog your pores.

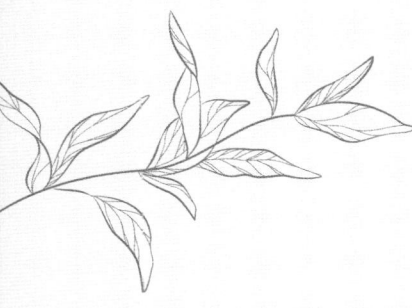

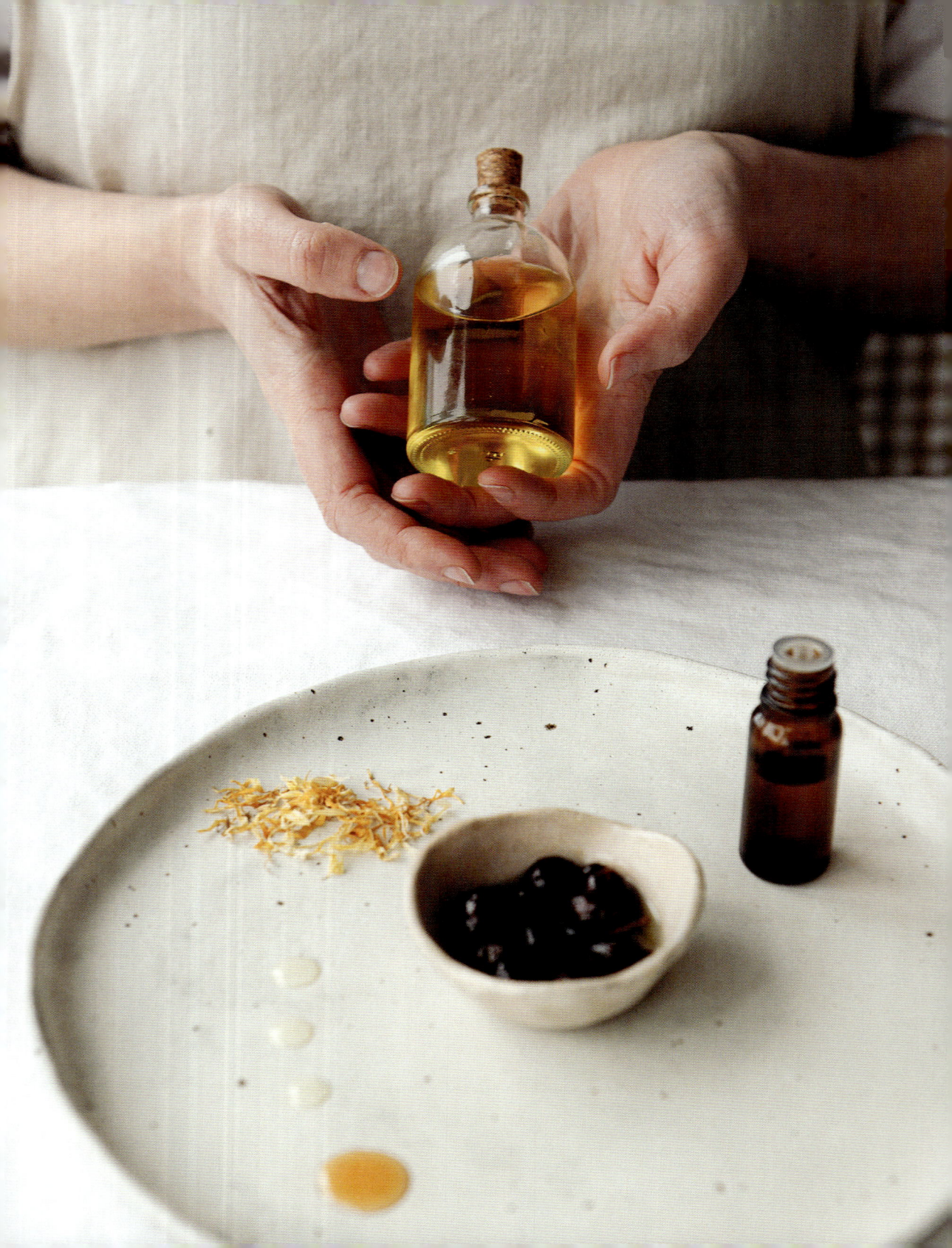

# GLOW FACE OIL

*I refer to this oil as "sunshine in a bottle." It is lovely and light and absorbs into your skin so quickly; the extra vitamin E and rosehip oils in this recipe are rich in antioxidants and anti-aging, and the apricot kernel oil is so lightweight and easily absorbed, helping it moisturize the skin without leaving a greasy feel. I love to use this throughout summer and particularly enjoy using it in the morning as it's softening and feels so refreshing on my skin.*

*Makes* 1 medium-sized bottle (100 ml [⅓ cup])

40 g (2½ tbsp) rosehip oil
28 g (2 tbsp) apricot kernel oil
20 g (1½ tbsp) jojoba oil
10 g (3 tsp) Calendula Infused Oil (page 120)
1.5 g vitamin E oil
0.5 g mandarin essential oil

Combine the rosehip oil, apricot kernel oil, jojoba oil and Calendula Infused Oil together in a bowl by stirring.

Add the vitamin E oil and mandarin essential oil and stir to combine.

Transfer to a sterile container.

Use two to three drops and massage into your face and neck to prepare your skin for the day.

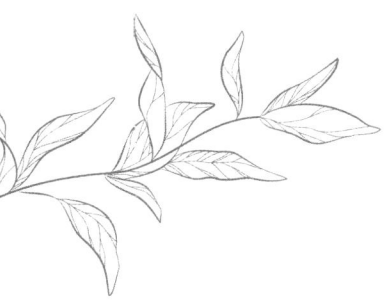

## Get to Know Your Ingredients!

This blend of oils will make your skin sing! You may notice that it is the first time I have used rosehip oil in a recipe in this book. It is rich in essential fatty acids and vitamins and is moisturizing, hydrating and softening. It is a heat-sensitive oil, which is why I have waited until this point to include it in a skin care recipe, as it would not respond well to recipes that require heat to create.

# RELAX AND RESTORE FACIAL OIL

*This is such a nourishing facial oil that can be used at any time of the day, but I particularly enjoy using it in the evening as part of my nighttime routine. It includes hemp seed oil, which again is the first time I have included this oil because it is heat sensitive and should only be used in cold infusion recipes. The jojoba oil in this recipe helps to regulate oil production and promotes skin health, while the hemp seed oil is a great source of omega 3 and omega 6 fatty acids and has anti-inflammatory properties.*

*Makes* 1 medium-sized bottle (100 ml [⅓ cup])

78 g (4½ tbsp) jojoba oil
10 g (3 tsp) hemp seed oil
10 g (3 tsp) Rosehip Infused Oil (page 128)
1.4 g vitamin E oil
0.3 g rosemary essential oil
0.3 g lavender essential oil

Combine the jojoba oil, hemp seed oil and Rosehip Infused Oil in a bowl by stirring.

Add the vitamin E oil, rosemary essential oil and lavender essential oil and stir again. Transfer to a sterile container for storing.

Rub two to three drops between the palms of your hands to release the aroma of the oils and deeply inhale the fragrance. Gently massage into your face and neck to soften, soothe and restore your skin.

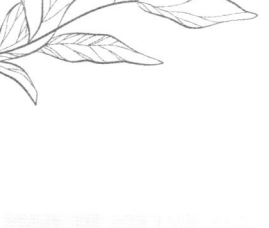

## Get to Know Your Ingredients!

For this restorative recipe, I have added hemp seed oil, which is both soothing and anti-inflammatory, and I have also added Rosehip Infused Oil, which is rich in vitamins and antioxidants. The essential oils I have included in this recipe are proven to fight stress and promote relaxation, making them a perfect nighttime ritual.

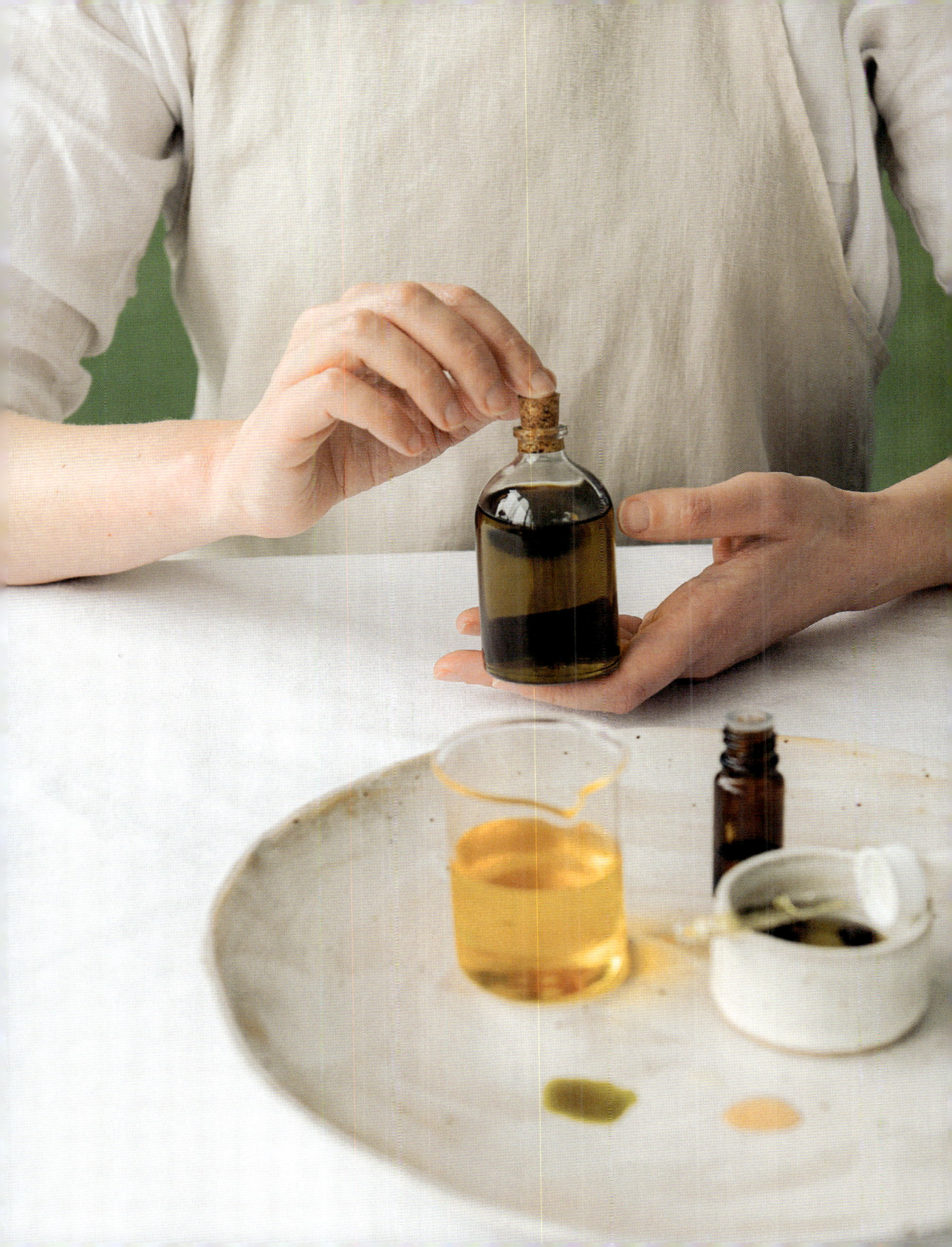

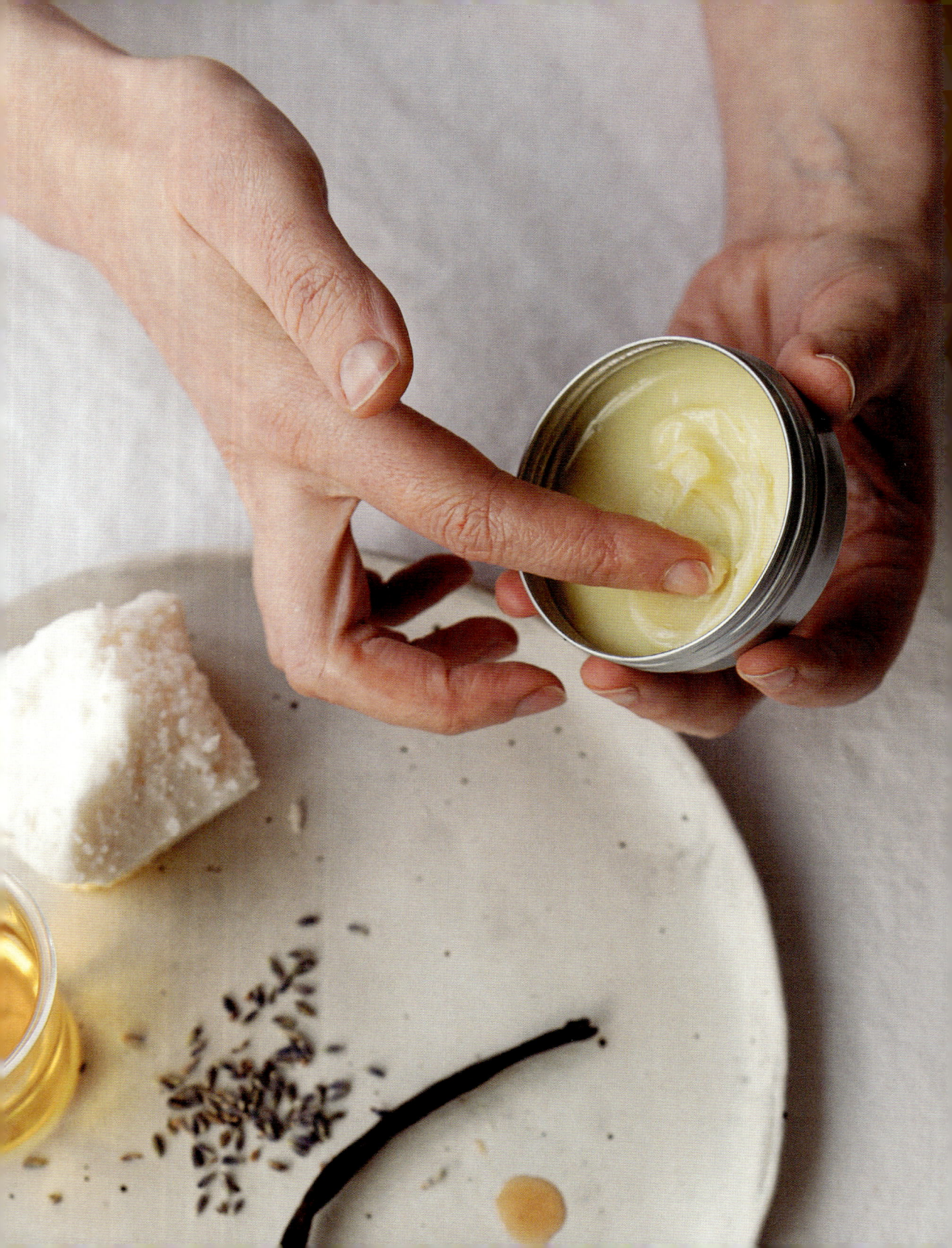

# NOURISHING JOJOBA FACE LOTION

*This is such an indulgent but gentle face lotion and is fantastic for treating tired, dry skin. I like to apply it at night before I fall asleep to wake up feeling hydrated and nourished. The ingredients are anti-aging, deeply moisturizing and rich in antioxidants, meaning your lotion will be working through the night to keep your skin feeling great.*

*Makes* 1 medium-sized jar
(100 g [½ cup])

40 g (2½ tbsp) jojoba oil

38 g (2½ tbsp) mango butter

10 g (3 tsp) Lavender Infused Oil (page 119)

10 g (3 tsp) Vanilla Pod Infused Oil (page 131)

2 g vitamin E oil

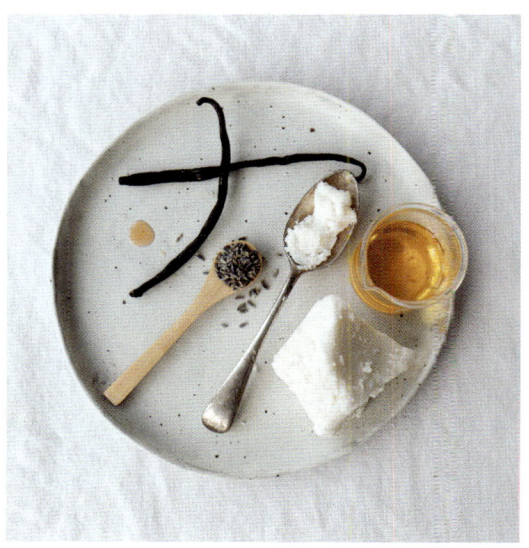

Using the double boiler method (read more about this on page 146), gently melt the jojoba oil, mango butter, Lavender Infused Oil and Vanilla Pod Infused Oil until it is a liquid consistency.

Place in the fridge, and when the mixture has cooled to below 105°F (40°C), add the vitamin E oil. This should take 10 to 15 minutes.

Allow the mixture to cool in the refrigerator until it solidifies. This should take approximately 1 hour.

Whip your mixture using a small electronic whisk (I use a frother-style whisk for this) for about 30 seconds until it is light and creamy. The mixture will become silky smooth.

Transfer to a clean, sterile container and allow to set for 24 hours. Massage a blueberry-sized amount into your skin for relaxation and hydration.

## Get to Know Your Ingredients!

Did you know that the composition of jojoba oil is similar to sebum, the natural oil produced by our skin's sebaceous glands? This makes it a fantastic addition to your skin care routine, as it helps to balance oil production and hydrate our skin without causing excessive oiliness. It is a great ingredient for all skin types, including oily and acne-prone skin.

# PROTECTIVE BALM

*This is the perfect treatment to protect your skin from cold weather and the dryness it brings. I love using this on my face, but it is a real all-purpose balm and is great for elbows, knees, lips—anywhere that needs a little extra care! This is a beautiful oil-in-balm formula, which transforms from a soft balm into a silky oil. The small amount of beeswax forms an occlusive layer on the skin and helps shield the skin from environmental stressors. I love to use this balm as a moisturizer throughout winter, as it leaves my skin feeling so soft and really protected. It is rich in antioxidants and high in vitamin E, which is a super anti-aging ingredient.*

*Makes* 1 medium-sized jar (100 g [½ cup])

50 g (3 tbsp) sweet almond oil

27 g (6 tsp) mango butter

10 g (3 tsp) Chamomile Flower Infused Oil (page 127)

5 g (1 tsp) beeswax

1 g vitamin E oil

Using the double boiler method, gently melt your sweet almond oil, mango butter, Chamomile Flower Infused Oil and beeswax until they are a liquid consistency. Read more about the double boiler method on page 146.

Take off the heat and place in the fridge.

When the mixture has cooled to below 105°F (40°C), add the vitamin E oil. This should take 10 to 15 minutes to cool. Stir to combine.

Allow the mixture to further cool in the fridge and stir as it cools until a trace line appears (read about trace lines on page 146). The trace line will appear quickly in this recipe.

Transfer to a clean, sterile container and allow to set overnight.

## Get to Know Your Ingredients!

If you do not want to use beeswax, then a great alternative is Candelilla wax. It has similar properties to the skin when used in skin care products and is also vegan friendly.

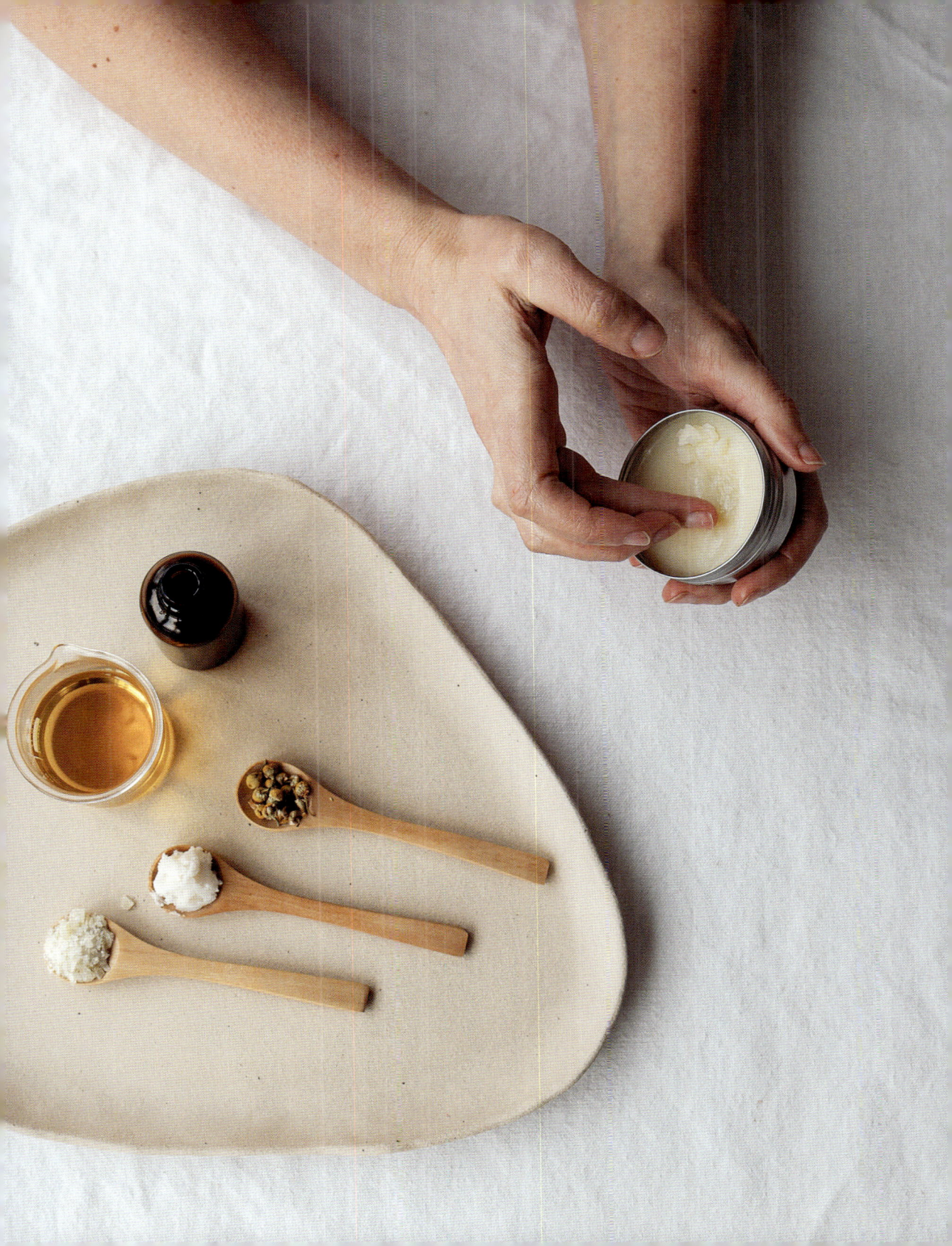

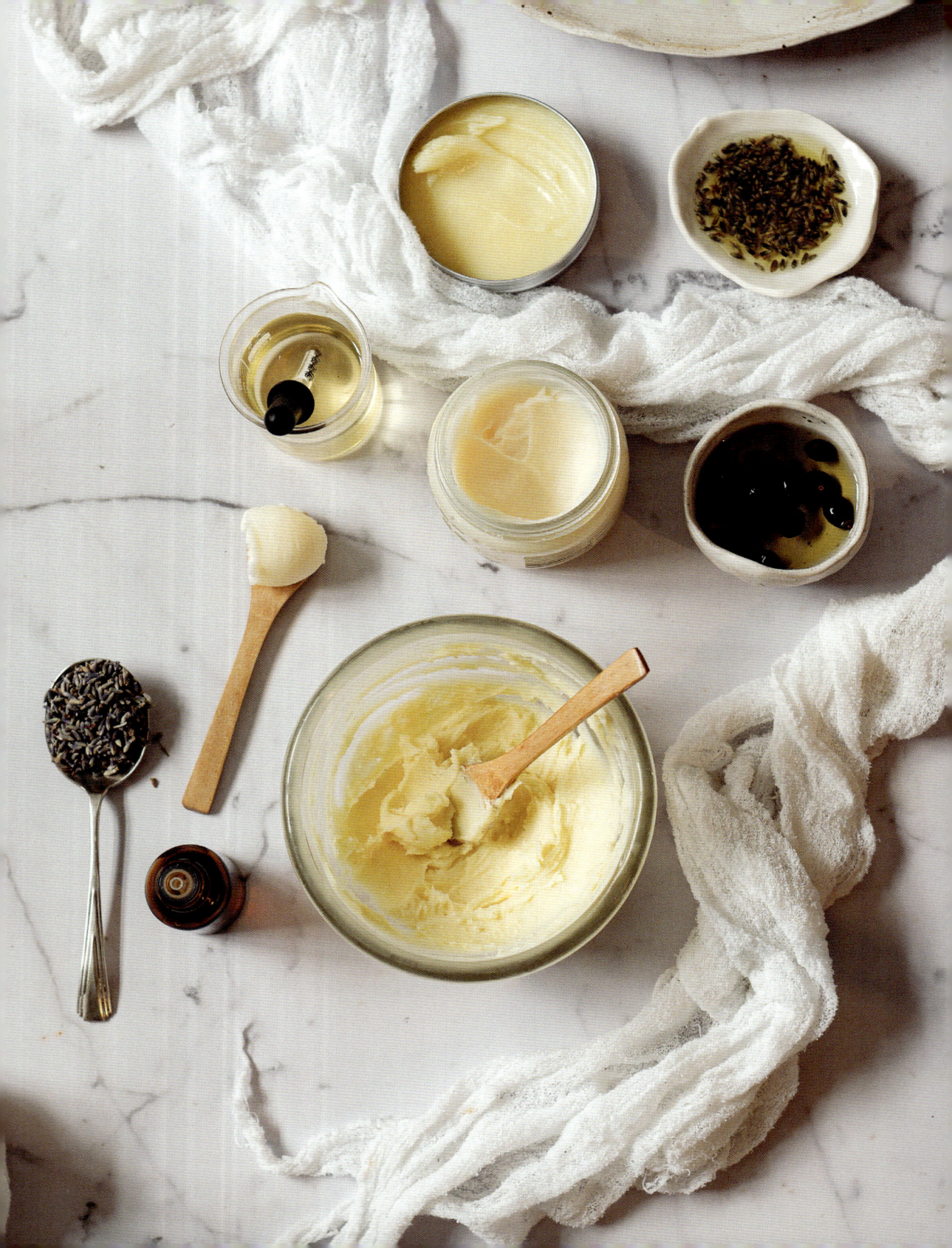

# BODY LOTIONS AND BUTTERS

I'm going to share some of my favorite body lotions and butters in this chapter. They are so exciting to make and are so unbelievably nourishing for your skin. I'll be sharing two different ways that I make them. The first way is super simple and creates a super smooth texture. The second way creates a texture like whipped cream and looks so good that you will want to eat it! These lotions and butters are jam-packed full of skin-loving ingredients that will leave your skin in tip-top condition.

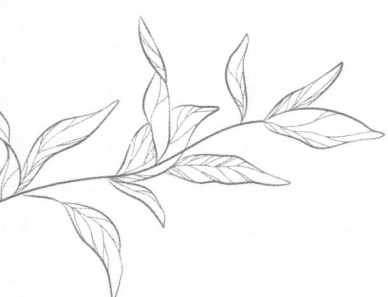

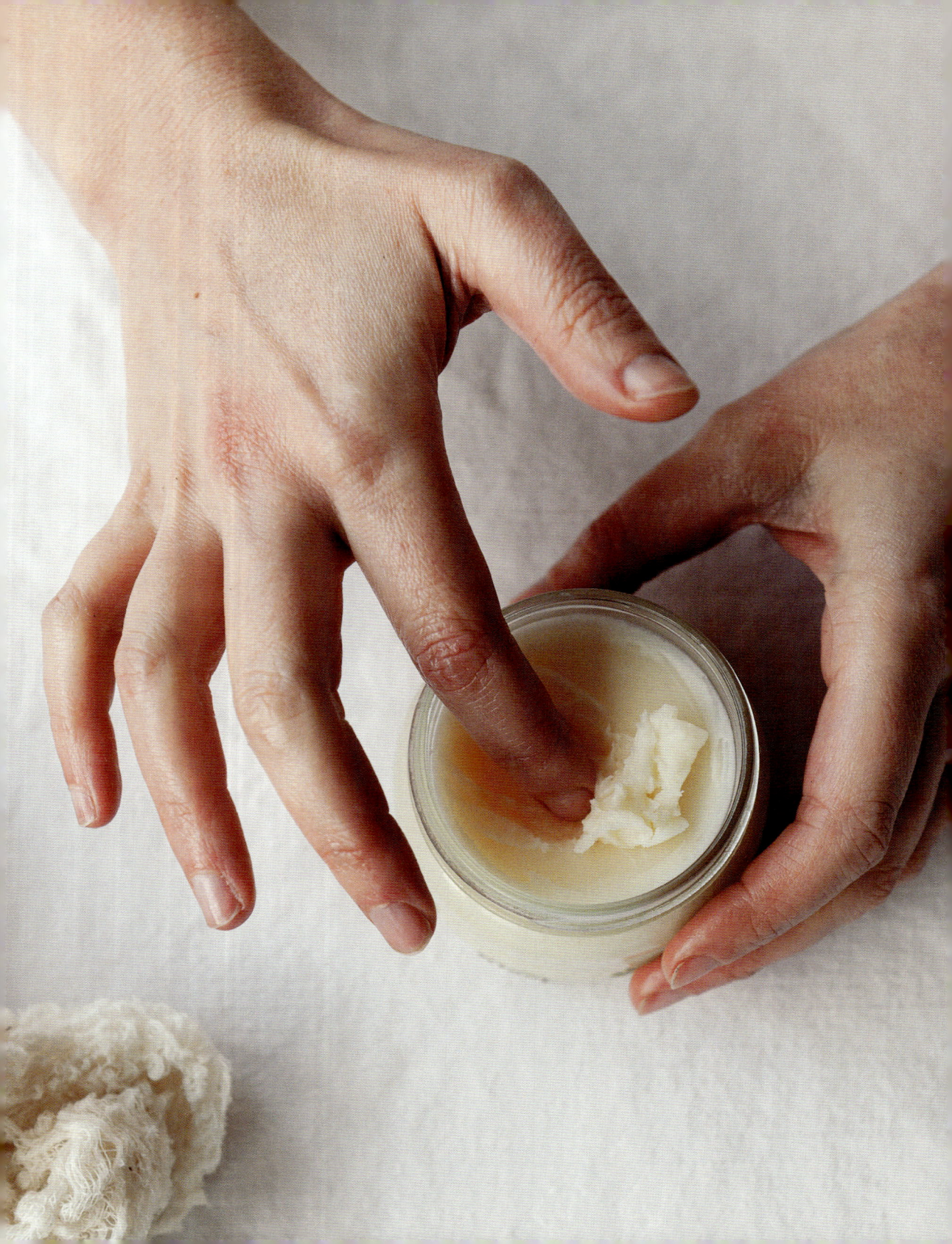

# NOURISHING VITAMIN E BODY LOTION

*Sometimes the simplest ingredients are the best! Whenever I whip up a batch of this lotion, I'm reminded of that. The consistency of the mango butter and sweet almond oil is light, and they sink into my skin quickly and easily . . . just lovely! This is one of the simplest recipes that I make, yet oh so indulgent at the same time. It combines three of my favorite ingredients (mango butter, sweet almond oil and vitamin E oil) to make the most gentle and soothing body lotion that is suitable for sensitive skin and it's anti-inflammatory.*

*Makes* 1 medium-sized jar (100 g [½ cup])

53 g (3 tbsp) sweet almond oil
45 g (10 tsp) mango butter
2 g vitamin E oil

Using the double boiler method (read more about performing this on page 146), gently melt the sweet almond oil and mango butter until it is of liquid consistency.

Place in the fridge and allow to cool. When the mixture has cooled to below 105°F (40°C), add the vitamin E oil. This should take 10 to 15 minutes to cool. Then, whisk the mixture.

Add to a clean, sterile container and place in the refrigerator to cool. Take it out and stir occasionally while it cools, until you see a trace line in the lotion. This should take between 30 to 60 minutes. See page 146 for more information on trace lines.

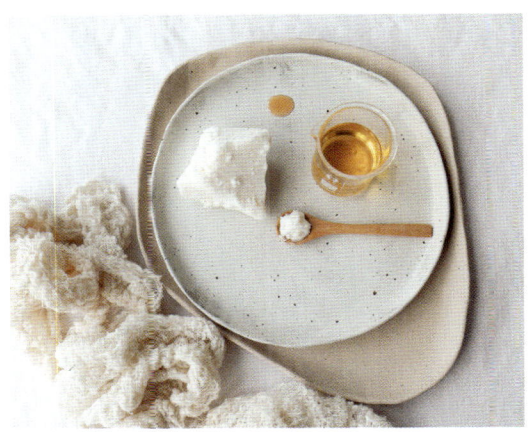

## Get to Know Your Ingredients!

You will notice that I include vitamin E in all of my recipes. Simply put, it is like a superfood for your skin and has so many benefits. Vitamin E is a powerful antioxidant, which helps prolong the shelf life of carrier oils and butters. Vitamin E also helps to protect the skin cells from damage caused by free radicals, which can cause premature aging, making it a great anti-aging addition to your skin care products.

# CALMING WHIPPED BODY BUTTER

*This is such a luxurious body butter and contains heaps of vitamin E. The texture is like whipped cream—it smells absolutely amazing and melts into your skin so quickly. I make double the quantity of this butter because all of my friends and family ask for some whenever I make it!*

*Makes* 1 large jar (200 g [1 cup])

99 g (6½ tbsp) mango butter

37 g (2½ tbsp) apricot kernel oil

30 g (2 tbsp) Vanilla Pod Infused Oil (page 131)

30 g (2 tbsp) Lavender Infused Oil (page 119)

4 g (1 tsp) vitamin E oil

Gently heat your mango butter, apricot kernel oil, Vanilla Pod Infused Oil and Lavender Infused Oil using a double boiler (read more about this method on page 146).

Take the mixture off the heat and allow to cool in the refrigerator.

When the mixture has cooled to below 105°F (40°C), add the vitamin E oil. This should take 10 to 15 minutes to cool.

Chill your mixture in the fridge until it becomes solid. This should take 1 to 2 hours.

Take your mixture out of the fridge, and using a handheld whisk, whisk until it becomes fluffy like whipped cream. This should only take 1 to 2 minutes, and you will see the color and texture of the butter change from a yellow solid to a light and fluffy cream. If the butter does not begin to change and instead stays quite liquid, then it didn't set for long enough in the fridge, so pop it back in for a little longer and repeat this step.

Add to a clean, sterile jar and store in a cool, dark place; you could even chill it in the fridge in warm weather.

## Get to Know Your Ingredients!

Lavender is such a healing botanical; it has antibacterial and anti-inflammatory properties, which means it is helpful in calming the skin and irritations on the skin. It has been reported that lavender is also good for minimizing the appearance of blemishes and scars.

Sweet almond oil is a popular oil that I always reach for. It is rich in squalene and vitamin E, which protect healthy cells from damage by free radicals. This oil is beneficial for all skin types, which makes it a great addition to your beauty kit.

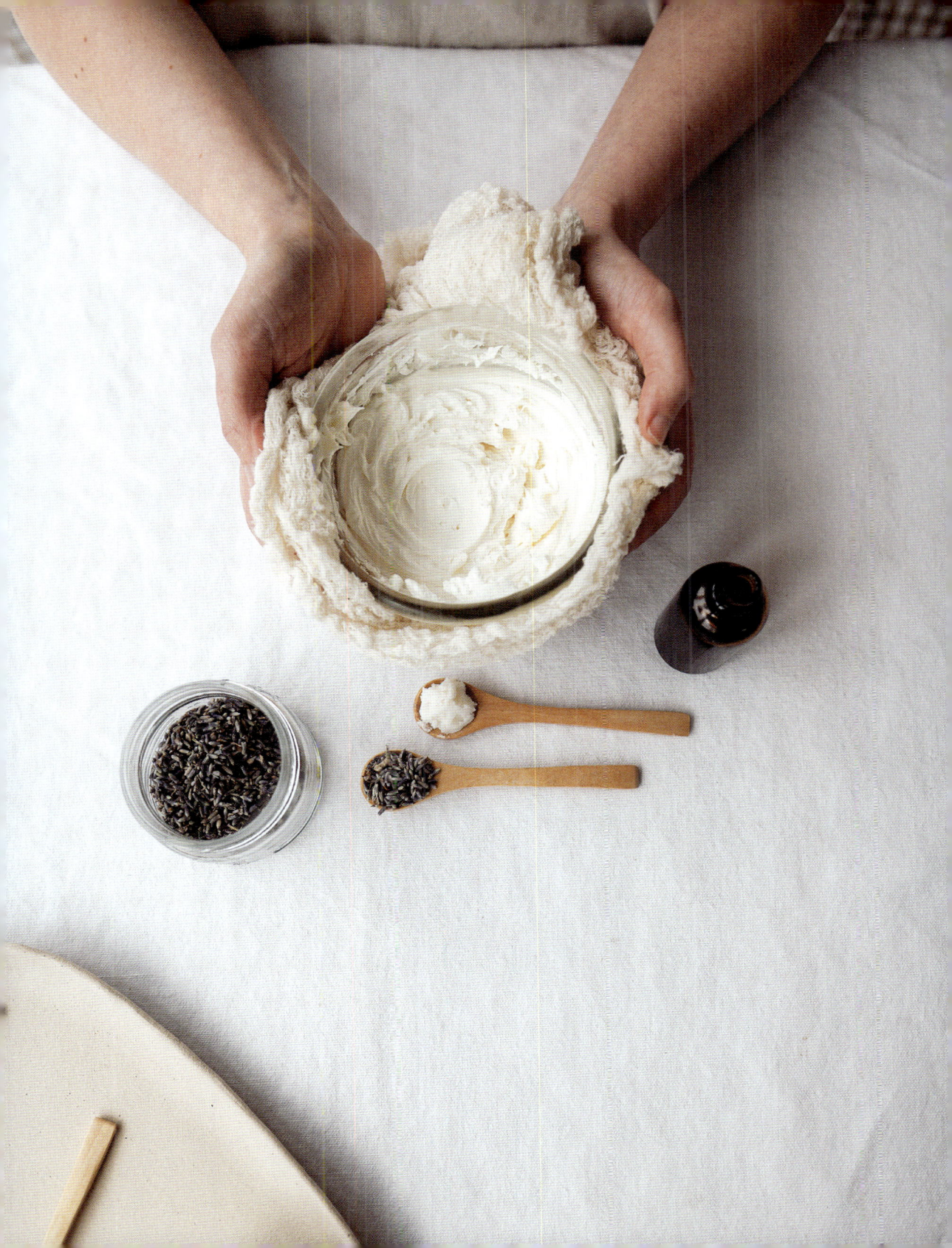

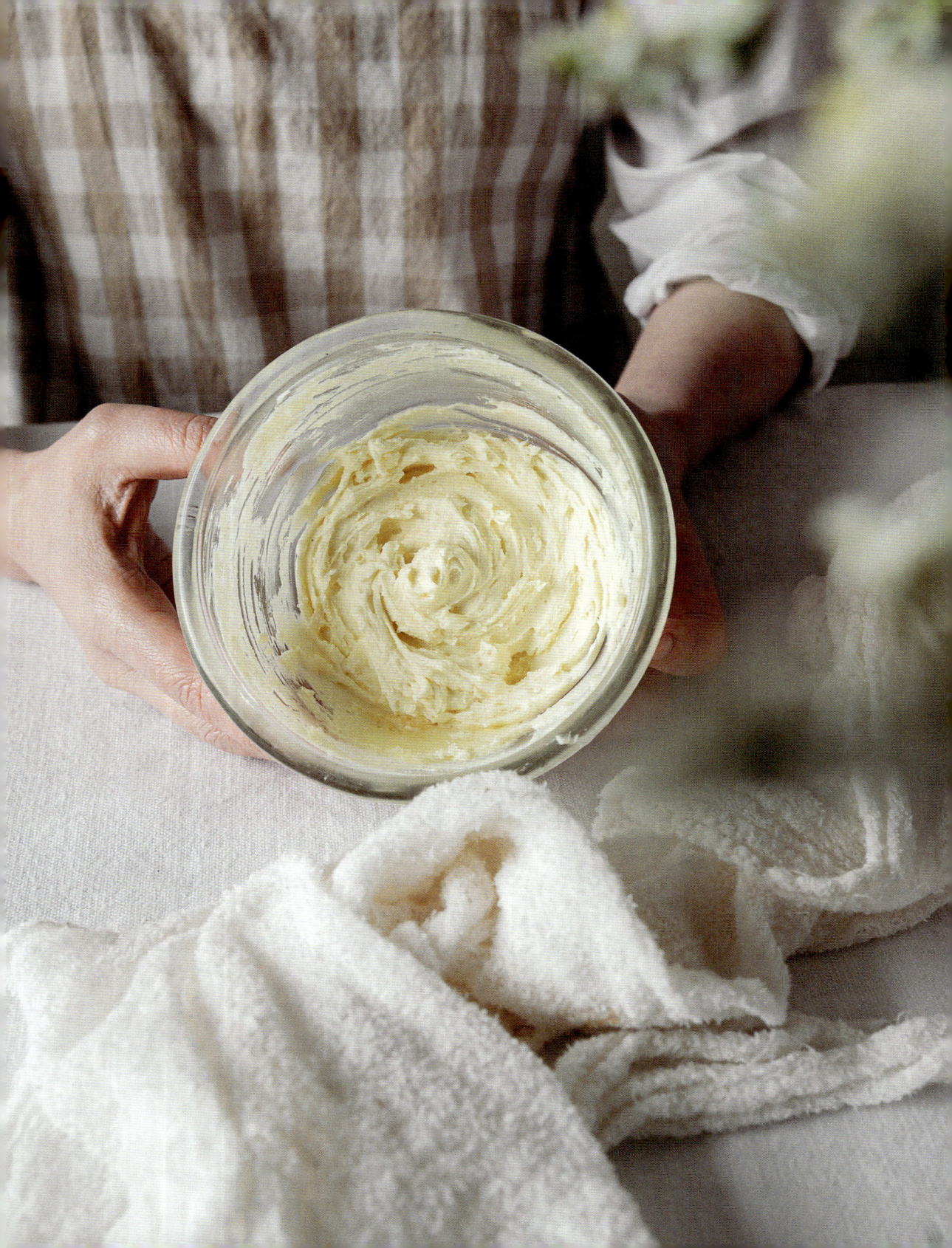

# BUTTERY BODY LOTION

*This lotion is a blend of beautiful butters and oils, which are whipped into a beautiful, rich lotion. The butters in this recipe are rich in essential fatty acids and are deeply moisturizing. The process of whipping the butters is so much fun. I recommend using this butter on those days that you feel your skin needs a little bit of extra care.*

*Makes* 1 medium-sized jar (100 g [½ cup])

28 g (2 tbsp) grapeseed oil

20 g (4 tsp) cocoa butter

20 g (1½ tbsp) shea butter

20 g (1½ tbsp) apricot kernel oil

10 g (3 tsp) Rose Petal Infused Oil (page 124)

1 g vitamin E oil

0.5 g chamomile essential oil

0.2 g geranium essential oil

0.3 g clary sage essential oil

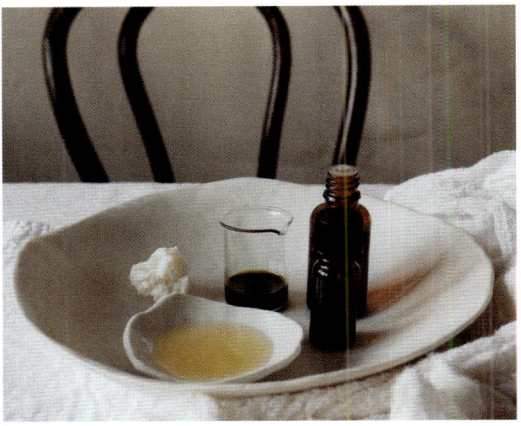

Using the double boiler method (read more about this method on page 146), gently melt the grapeseed oil, cocoa butter, shea butter, apricot kernel oil and Rose Petal Infused Oil until it is a liquid consistency.

Place in the fridge and allow the mixture to cool.

When the mixture has cooled to below 105°F (40°C), add the vitamin E oil, chamomile essential oil, geranium essential oil and clary sage essential oil. This should take 10 to 15 minutes to cool. Then whisk the mixture.

Add to a clean, sterile jar and place in the refrigerator to cool further. Take it out and stir occasionally while it cools, until you see a trace line in the lotion. This should take between 30 to 60 minutes. See page 146 for more information on trace lines.

Store in a cool, dark place; you could even chill it in the fridge in warm weather.

## Get to Know Your Ingredients!

I have used Rose Petal Infused Oil for this recipe; it is a beautiful ingredient for those of us with dry and sensitive skin and is known for its brightening properties. In addition to this, I have added essential oils, which really complement the butters, aid in relaxation and turn your moisturizing routine into a mindfulness routine, as the aroma will help you relax as you gently massage it into your skin.

# INDULGENT WHIPPED BODY BUTTER

*The final butter that I am sharing is another beautifully whipped butter that smells heavenly while also being super gentle on your skin. The butter is rich in vitamins A and E and promotes skin elasticity. It is the perfect butter to enjoy as part of your skin care routine to keep your skin smooth and supple.*

*Makes* 1 large jar (200 g [1 cup])

98 g (6½ tbsp) mango butter

90 g (5 tbsp) jojoba oil

10 g (3 tsp) Calendula Infused Oil (page 120)

1 g vitamin E

0.5 g rosemary essential oil

0.5 g mandarin essential oil

0.2 g clove essential oil

Gently heat your mango butter, jojoba oil and Calendula Infused Oil using the double boiler method until it is a liquid consistency (read more about this method on page 146).

Take off the heat and place in the refrigerator to cool. When the mixture has cooled to below 77°F (25°C), add the vitamin E oil, rosemary essential oil, mandarin essential oil and clove essential oil and stir to combine.

Chill your mixture in the fridge until it becomes solid. This should take about 1 hour.

Take your mixture out of the fridge, and using a handheld whisk, whisk until it becomes fluffy. This should only take 1 to 2 minutes, and you will see the color and texture of the butter change from a solid yellow to a light and fluffy cream. If the butter does not begin to change and instead stays quite liquid, then it didn't set for long enough in the fridge, so pop it back in for a little longer and repeat this step.

Add to a clean, sterile jar.

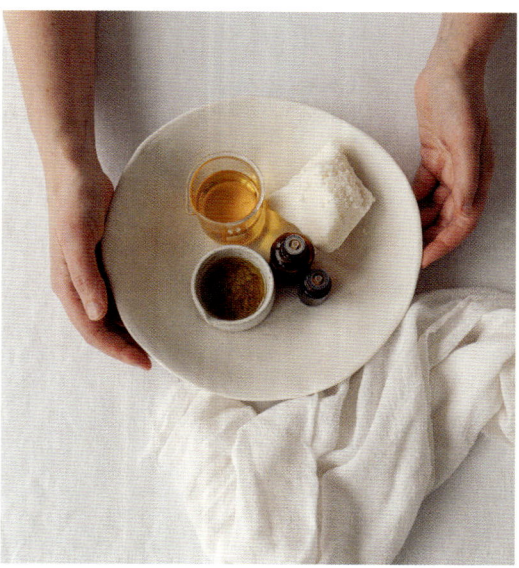

### Get to Know Your Ingredients!

Calendula has been used in herbal medicine for centuries because of its many health benefits. It has anti-inflammatory and antioxidant properties and helps to soothe and calm irritated skin, making it a beautiful addition to this indulgent whipped body butter.

The blend of essential oils in this recipe is woody and citrusy, giving this lotion a wonderfully indulgent aroma.

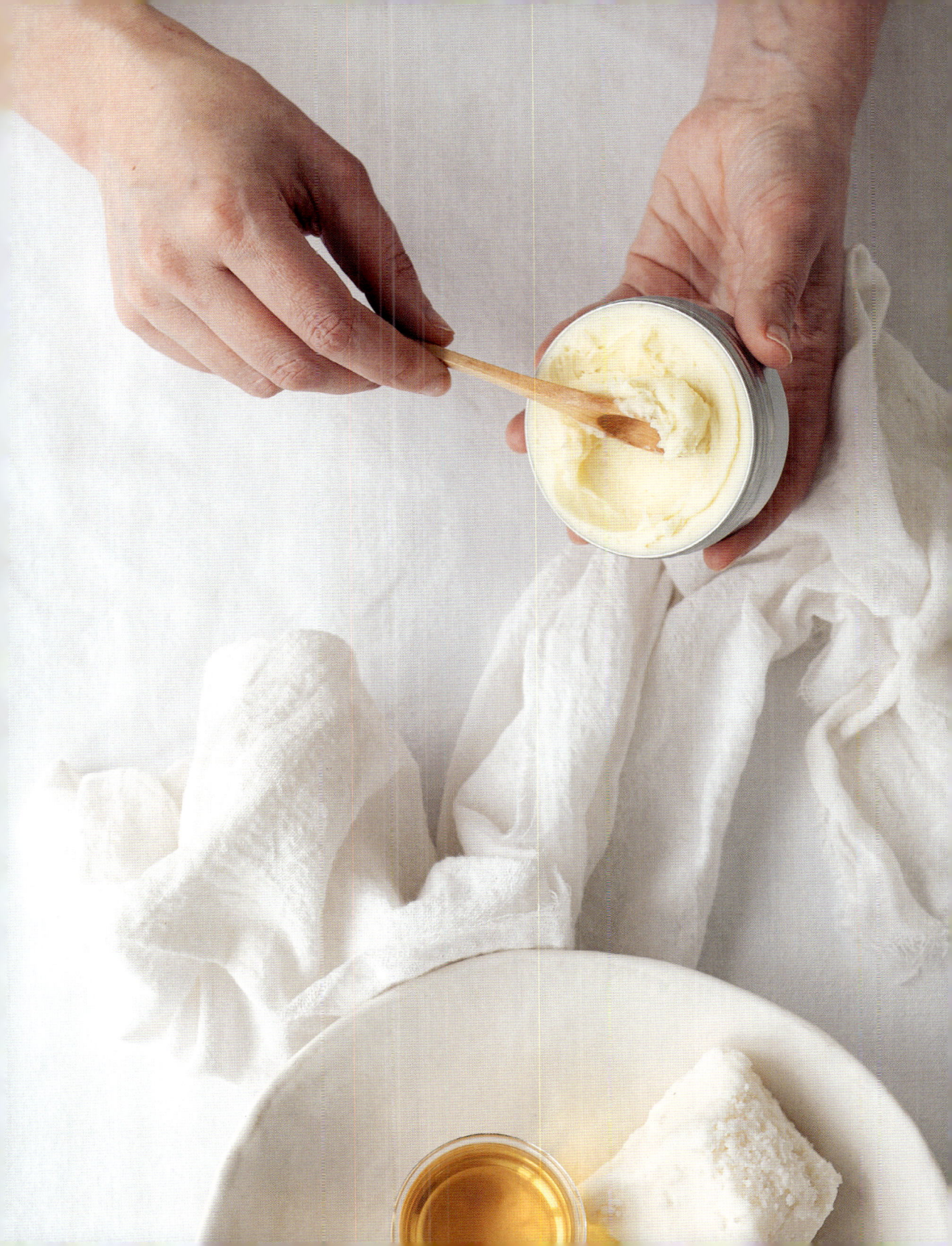

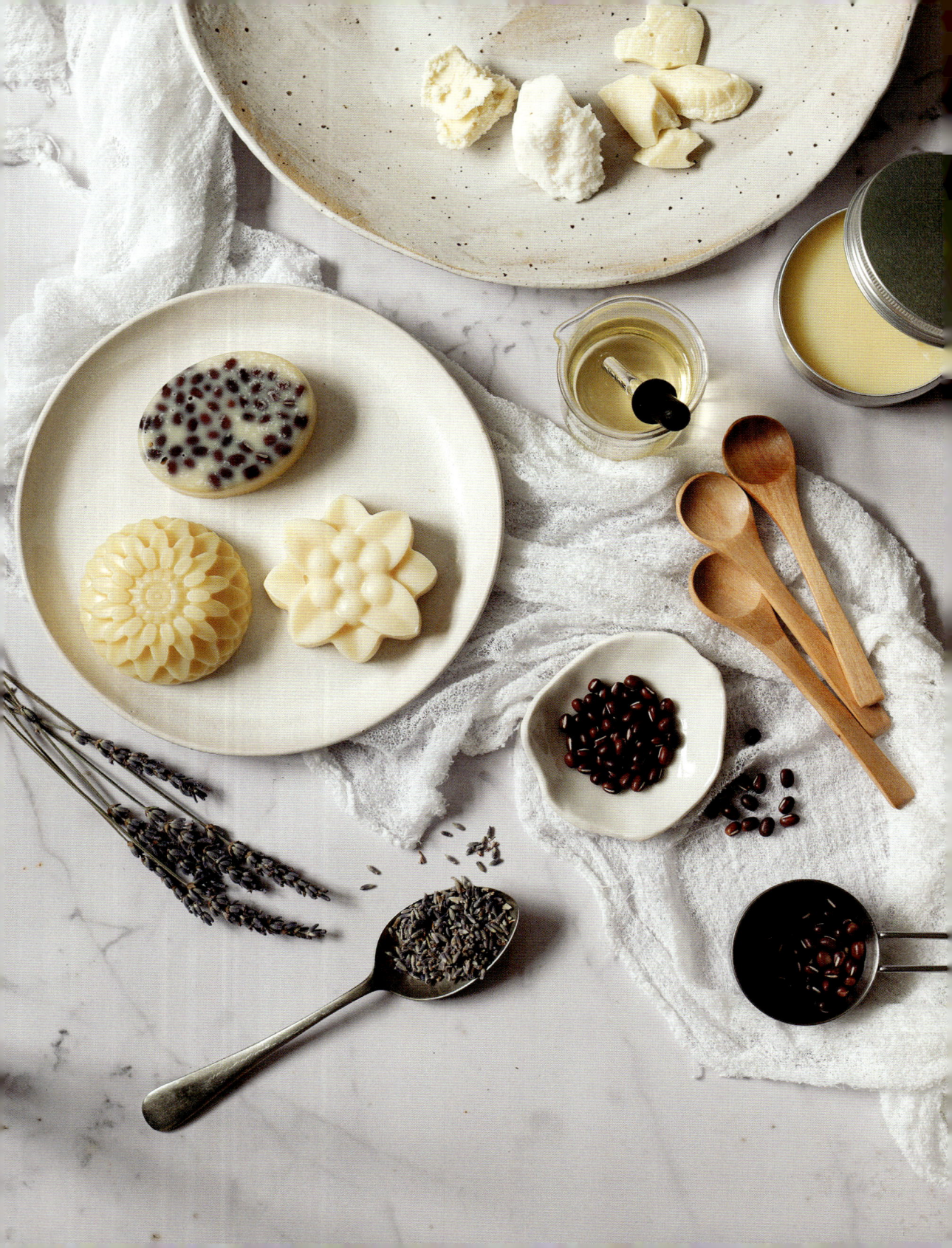

# LOTION BARS

I have a bit of a love affair with beauty products in bar form and have loved massage bars for many years. Massage bars are so soothing and are thought to help your muscles recover faster by helping to release tension and soreness when they are rubbed into your skin. I have also included a massage balm, which is a beautiful solid consistency that quickly melts into your skin. I use silicone molds in these recipes to help create the lotion bars. They are quite easy to find and really you can use any shape depending on your preference. If you don't have silicone molds and would prefer to use something that you have in the kitchen cupboard, a great alternative is to simply use a muffin tin to create the shape.

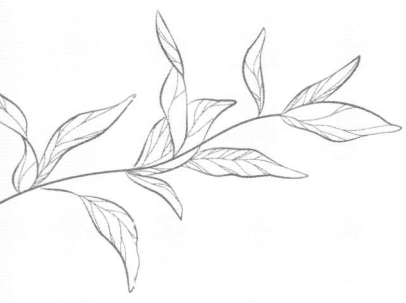

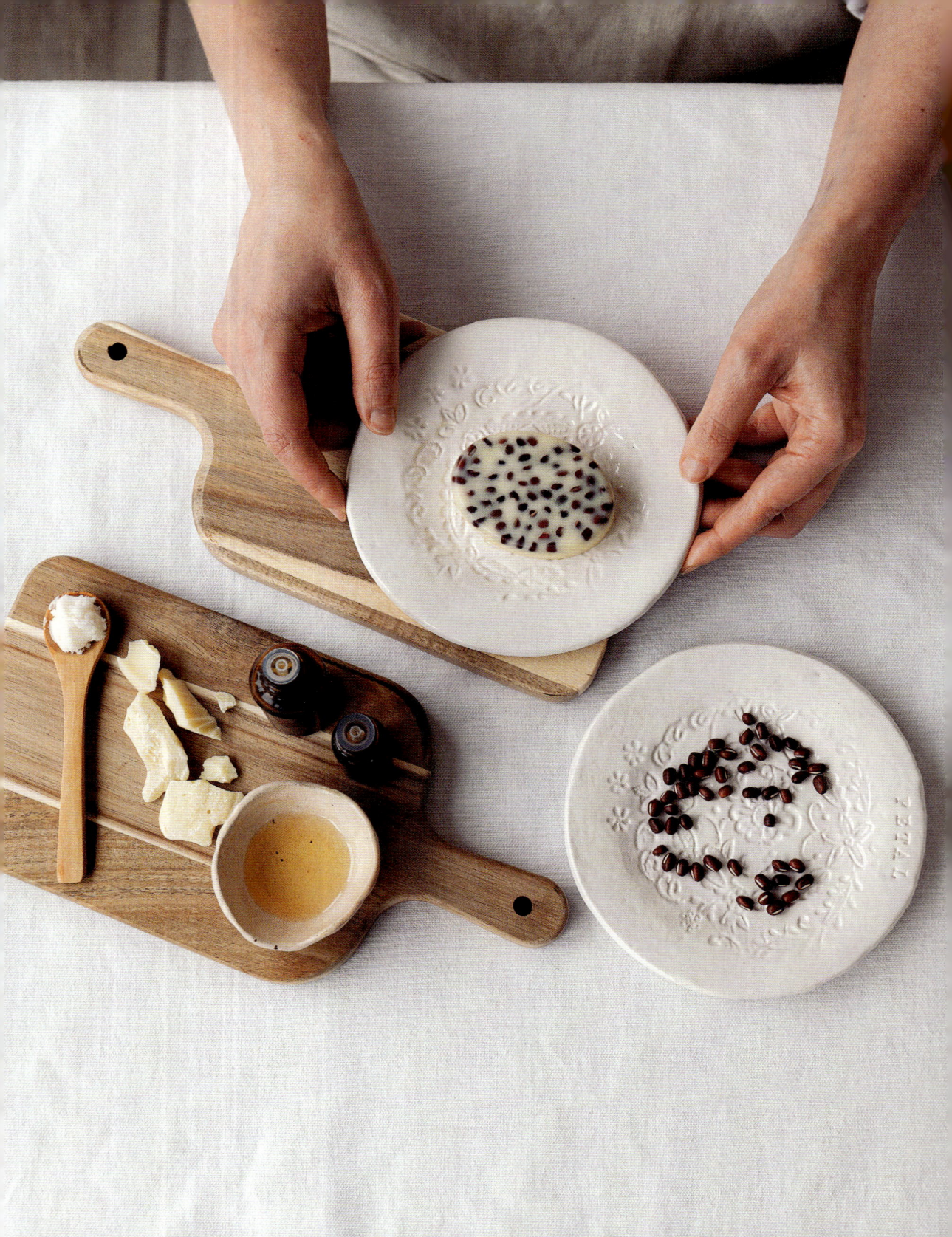

# DEEP MUSCLE MASSAGING BAR

*I love using these bars to massage my tired muscles. This bar is naturally rich in vitamin E, which helps to soften and smooth your skin, and the adzuki beans help to work away any tensions. Massage the bar into your dry skin and it will soon be nourished and refreshed thanks to the bar's skin-conditioning butters and oils.*

*Makes* 2 medium-sized bars

55 g (12 tsp) cocoa butter

18 g (4 tsp) mango butter

5 g (1 tsp) sweet almond oil

20 g (¼ cup) adzuki beans

1 g vitamin E oil

1 g mandarin essential oil

Gently heat the cocoa butter, mango butter and sweet almond oil using the double boiler method until they are fully combined and a liquid consistency. Read more about using the double boiler method on page 146.

Once melted, take off the heat, add the adzuki beans and allow to cool. When the mixture has cooled to 77°F (25°C), add the vitamin E oil and mandarin essential oil and whisk to combine. This should take 10 to 15 minutes to cool.

Add the mixture to the mold of your choice and chill overnight in the fridge. I like to use oval ones, as they fit nicely in the palm of my hand.

Massage into your skin for a deep and soothing massage.

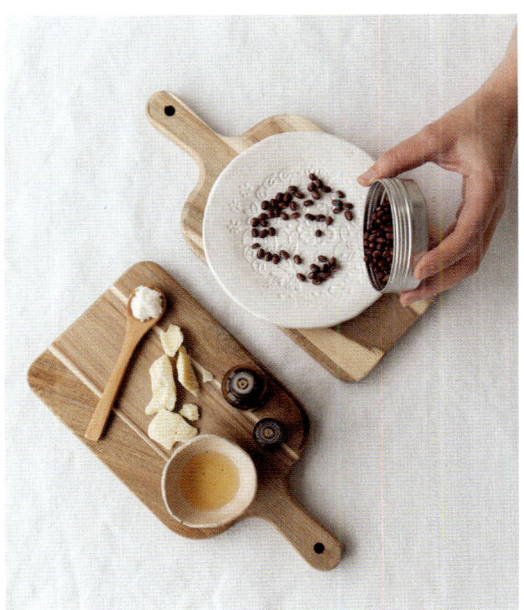

### Get to Know Your Ingredients!

Cocoa butter helps improve skin elasticity and is great for dry skin. It has a low melting point, which makes it ideal to be used in lotion bars, as the butter melts when in contact with warm skin. The mandarin essential oil smells beautiful in this bar and also helps to reduce inflammation and complements the cocoa butter beautifully.

# RELAXING MASSAGE LOTION BAR

*I have made this massage bar with a lovely blend of essential oils that helps to promote calm and relaxation. I have also included softer butters in this recipe. You will notice that this means the lotion bar melts differently when rubbed over your skin, and I find that it is absorbed into my skin quite rapidly. If you live in a warmer climate, it may be useful to keep this bar in the fridge between uses, as it will have a lower melting point than cocoa butter alone.*

*Makes* 2 medium-sized bars

55 g (12 tsp) cocoa butter
28 g (2 tbsp) shea butter
10 g (1 tbsp) mango butter
5 g (1 tsp) sweet almond oil
1 g vitamin E oil
0.4 g lavender essential oil
0.4 g mandarin essential oil
0.2 g clove essential oil

Gently heat the cocoa butter, shea butter, mango butter and sweet almond oil using the double boiler method (see page 146 for more information) until they are fully combined and a liquid consistency.

Once liquid, take the mixture off the heat and place in the refrigerator. Wait for the mixture to cool to below 77°F (25°C), then add the vitamin E oil, lavender essential oil, mandarin essential oil and clove essential oil. This should take 10 to 15 minutes to cool.

Add the mixture to the mold of your choice and chill overnight in the fridge.

These bars should last 3 months and are shelf-stable.

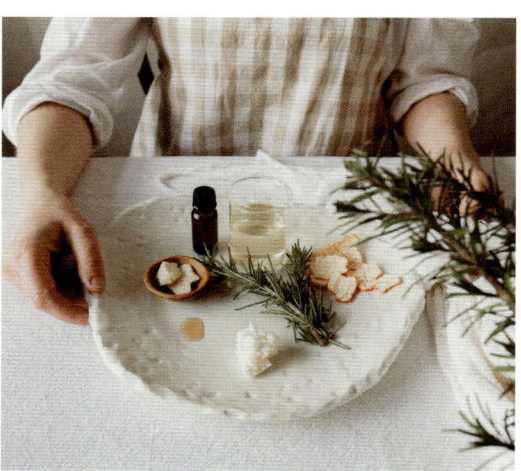

## Get to Know Your Ingredients!

This is a beautiful lotion bar that provides just the right mixture of massage and aromatherapy to help you relax. I have added shea butter to this lotion bar, so that you can understand the differences between butters and how they work on the skin. Shea butter is a softer butter than cocoa butter and melts differently when in contact with skin. It's interesting to find which butter you prefer to use!

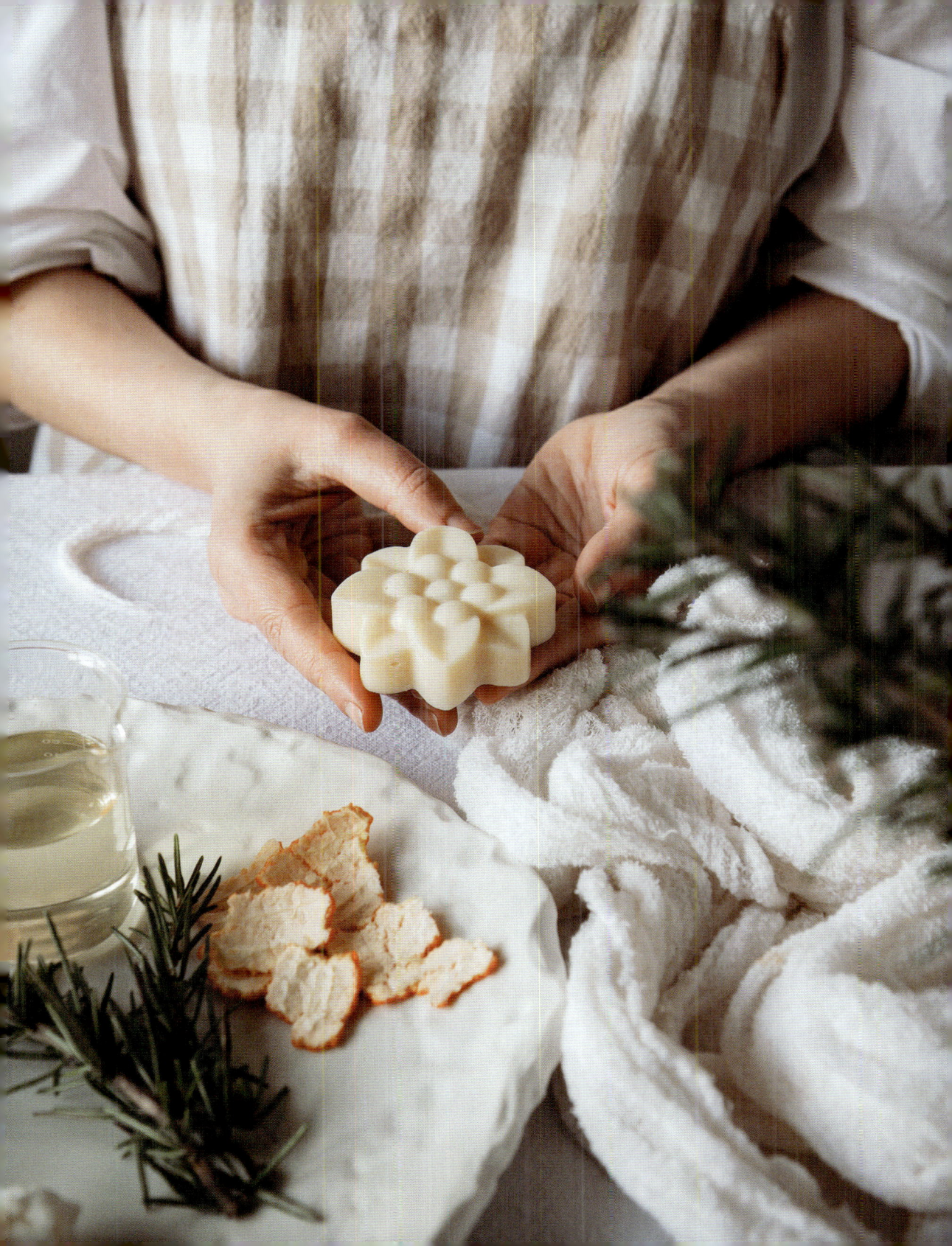

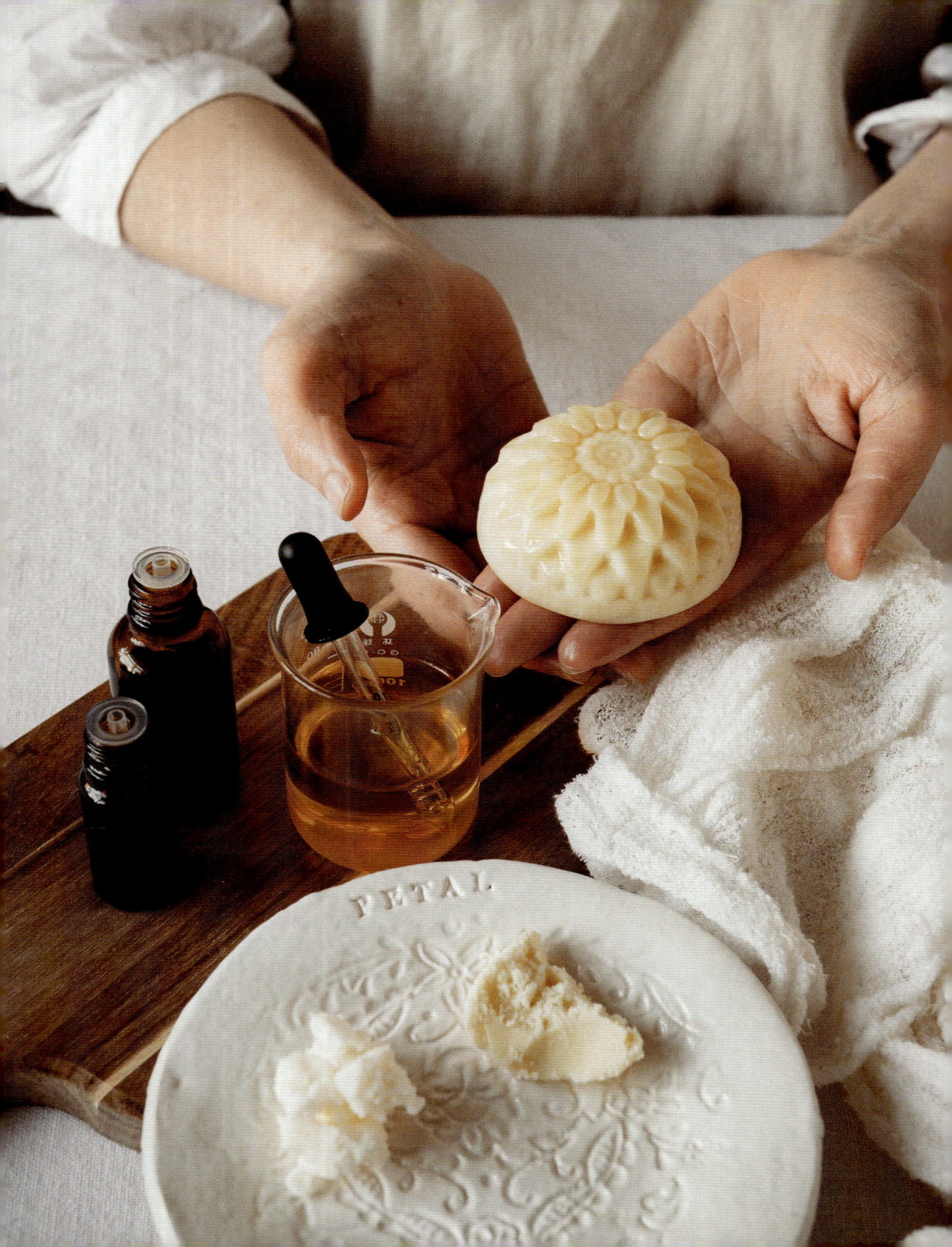

# EVERYDAY RITUALS MASSAGING LOTION BAR

*I love using this lotion bar as part of my morning routine. The eucalyptus, mandarin and rosemary feel really refreshing and also help to improve my mental focus, which is a necessity for this tired mum! As it is a lotion bar, I massage it into my body to help boost my circulation, nourish my skin and prepare me for the day.*

*Makes* 2 medium-sized bars

50 g (10 tsp) cocoa butter
38 g (2½ tbsp) shea butter
10 g (3 tsp) sweet almond oil
1 g vitamin E oil
0.5 g mandarin essential oil
0.3 g rosemary essential oil
0.2 g eucalyptus essential oil

Gently heat the cocoa butter, shea butter and sweet almond oil using the double boiler method until they are fully combined and a liquid consistency. Read more about using the double boiler method on page 146.

Take off the heat, place in the refrigerator and allow the mixture to cool to below 77°F (25°C), then add the vitamin E oil, mandarin essential oil, rosemary essential oil and eucalyptus essential oil and mix together. This should take 10 to 15 minutes to cool.

Add to the mold of your choice and chill overnight in the fridge.

If you live in a warmer climate, it may be a good idea to refrigerate your bars so that they do not melt before you use them.

## Get to Know Your Ingredients!

This lotion bar is deeply moisturizing and a natural emollient, which helps to soften and smooth the skin. The eucalyptus essential oil that I have used in this bar also has anti-inflammatory properties, which can help to soothe irritated skin and prepare your skin for the day.

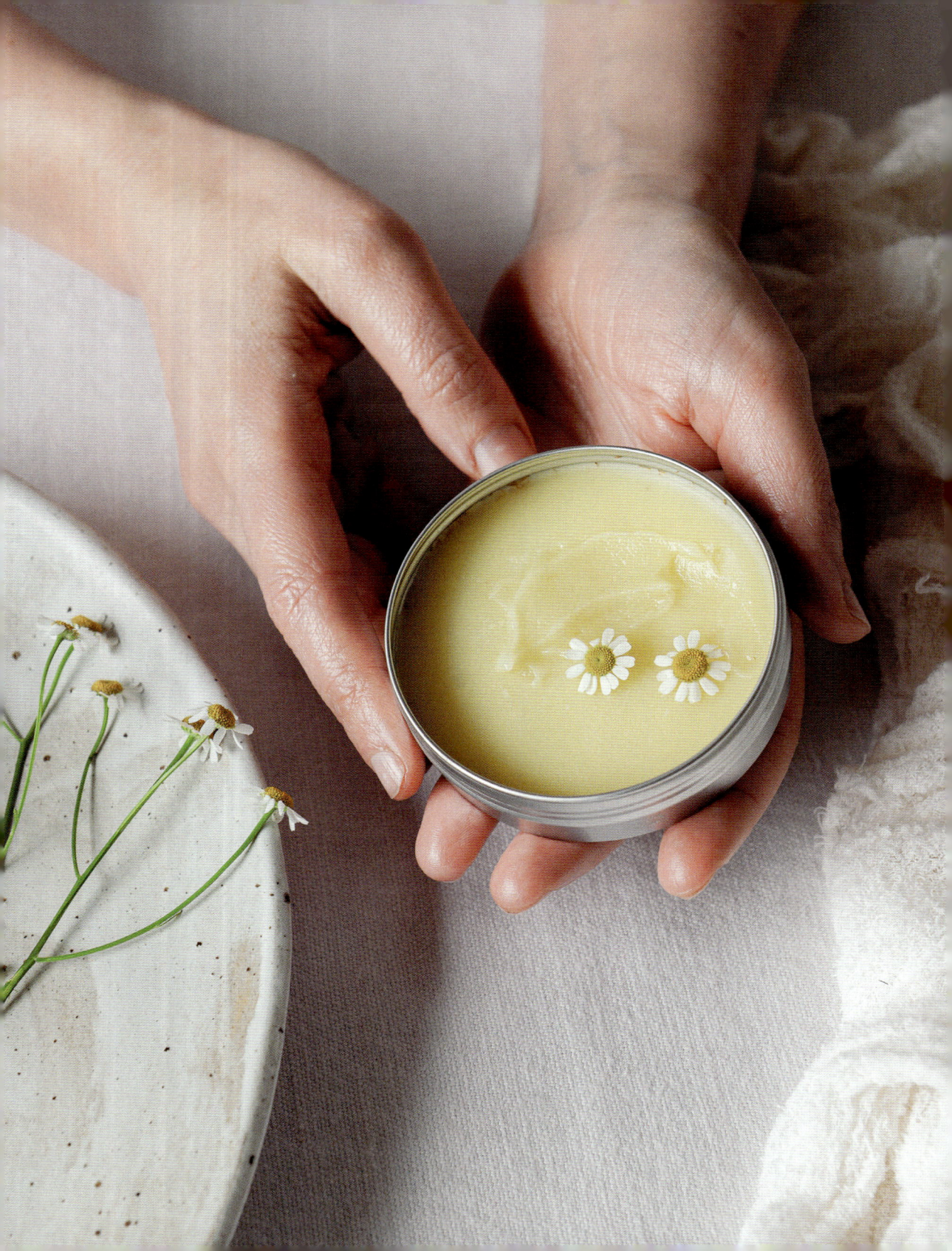

# BALMS

I'm sharing some of my favorite nourishing balm recipes to help heal and hydrate the skin in this chapter, beginning with my favorite go-to balm for those long sunny days when your skin feels like it needs extra care. The blend of ingredients I use in balms has been chosen to be intensely nourishing and help to promote healing and also soothe dry, chapped skin. Balms are also a fantastic addition for mature skin. Many of my family members use these balms year round in place of a moisturizer, and I also switch to them in winter for an extra layer of protection. They are a hero product!

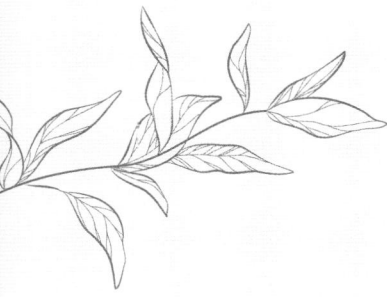

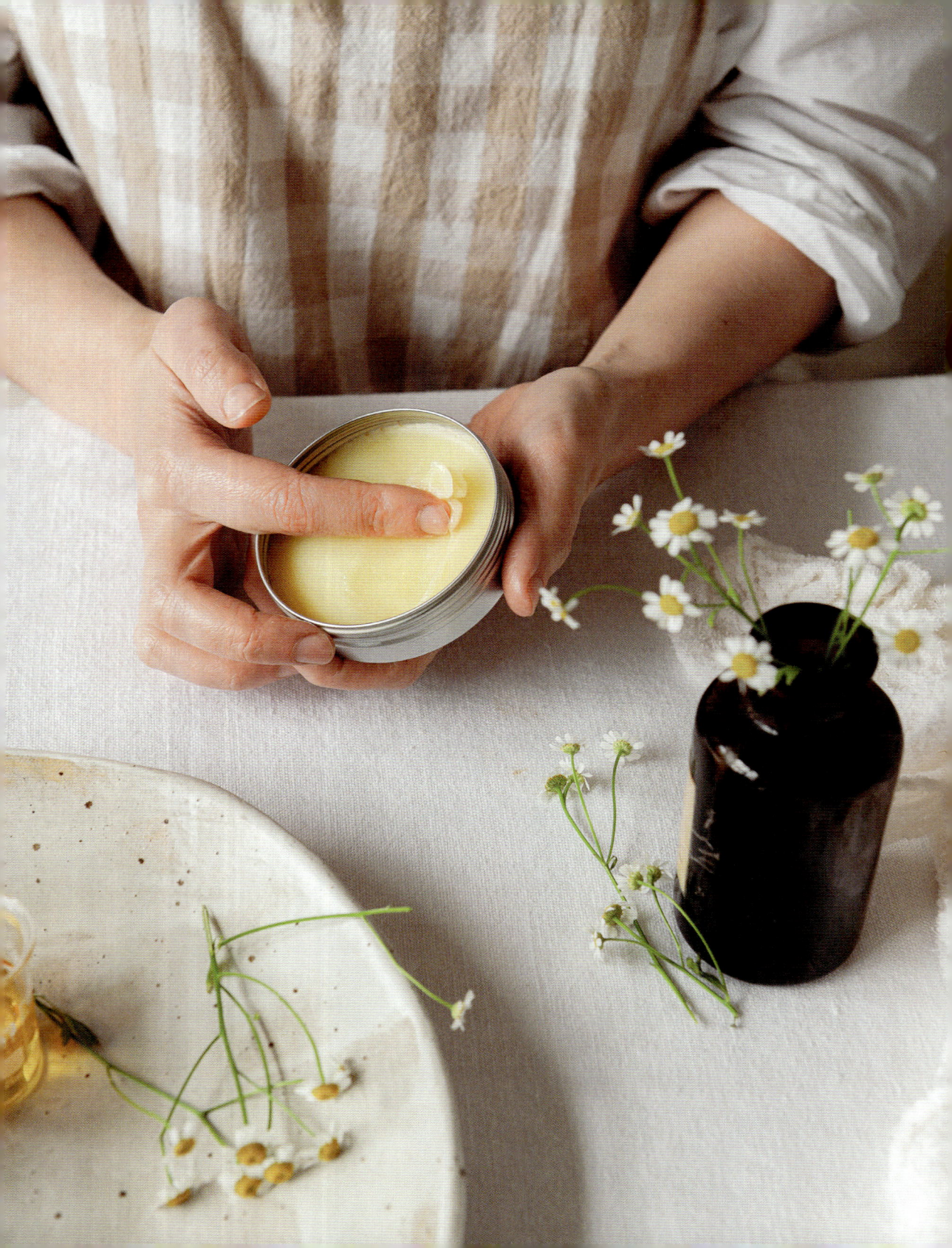

# AFTER-SUN SOOTHING BALM

*I have created this as quite a soft balm that you can scoop out if you need a good amount. You can also store it in the fridge for a more solid balm if you prefer. The ingredients used in this balm are skin healing, calming and soothing, perfect to treat your skin with a little love.*

*Makes* 1 medium-sized tin (100 g [4 oz])

27 g (2 tbsp) shea butter
25 g (2 tbsp) jojoba oil
25 g (2 tbsp) sweet almond oil
10 g (3 tsp) Calendula Infused Oil (page 120)
5 g (1 tsp) beeswax
1 g vitamin E oil
1 g chamomile essential oil

Gently melt the shea butter, jojoba oil, sweet almond oil, Calendula Infused Oil and beeswax using the double boiler method (read more about this on page 146).

Take off the heat and place in the refrigerator. This should take 10 to 15 minutes to cool.

When the mixture reaches below 77°F (25°C), add the vitamin E oil and chamomile essential oil. Blend together and transfer to a sterile container. I find a shallow tin works well for this formula.

Allow to set for 24 hours before using.

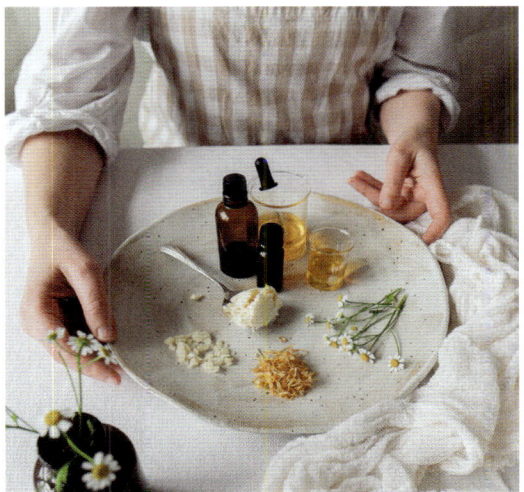

## Get to Know Your Ingredients!

Shea butter is well-known for its moisturizing properties and is rich in oleic acid, which helps to replenish the skin's lipid barrier, preventing water loss and keeping the skin hydrated.

Additionally, calendula and chamomile provide further support as after-sun products, as they both contain anti-inflammatory compounds, antibacterial properties and antioxidants, which protect the skin from free radicals.

# BOTANICAL BRUISE BALM

*I have used this bruise balm for years, and it is just amazing at helping to reduce bruises and promote faster healing. It is a perfect ointment for my children too! In the winter, I make this using chamomile (which I will show you in this recipe), but in the summer, I collect daisies to create this balm!*

*Makes* 1 medium-sized tin (100 g [4 oz])

43 g (2½ tbsp) sweet almond oil

20 g (1½ tbsp) beeswax

35 g (2 tbsp) Chamomile Flower Infused Oil (page 127)

1 g vitamin E oil

Using the double boiler method, melt the sweet almond oil, beeswax and Chamomile Flower Infused Oil until they are a liquid consistency. Read more about the double boiler method on page 146.

When the mixture becomes a liquid consistency, add to the fridge. When the mixture cools below 77°F (25°C), add the vitamin E oil. This should take 10 to 15 minutes to cool.

Add to a sterile container and allow to cool and set in the fridge overnight.

Apply to bumps and bruises as needed!

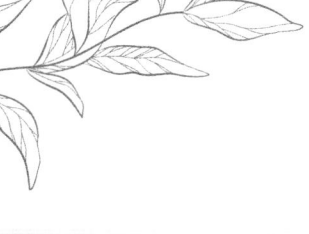

## Get to Know Your Ingredients!

Did you know that the common daisy (also known as bellis perennis) has been used in traditional medicine for years for its wound-healing properties to aid in the recovery of minor cuts and bruises? I pick them straight from my garden and dry them out to make this blended oil. If you do not have daisies available where you live or they aren't in season, you could substitute for chamomile, which is a lovely botanical that shares similar properties.

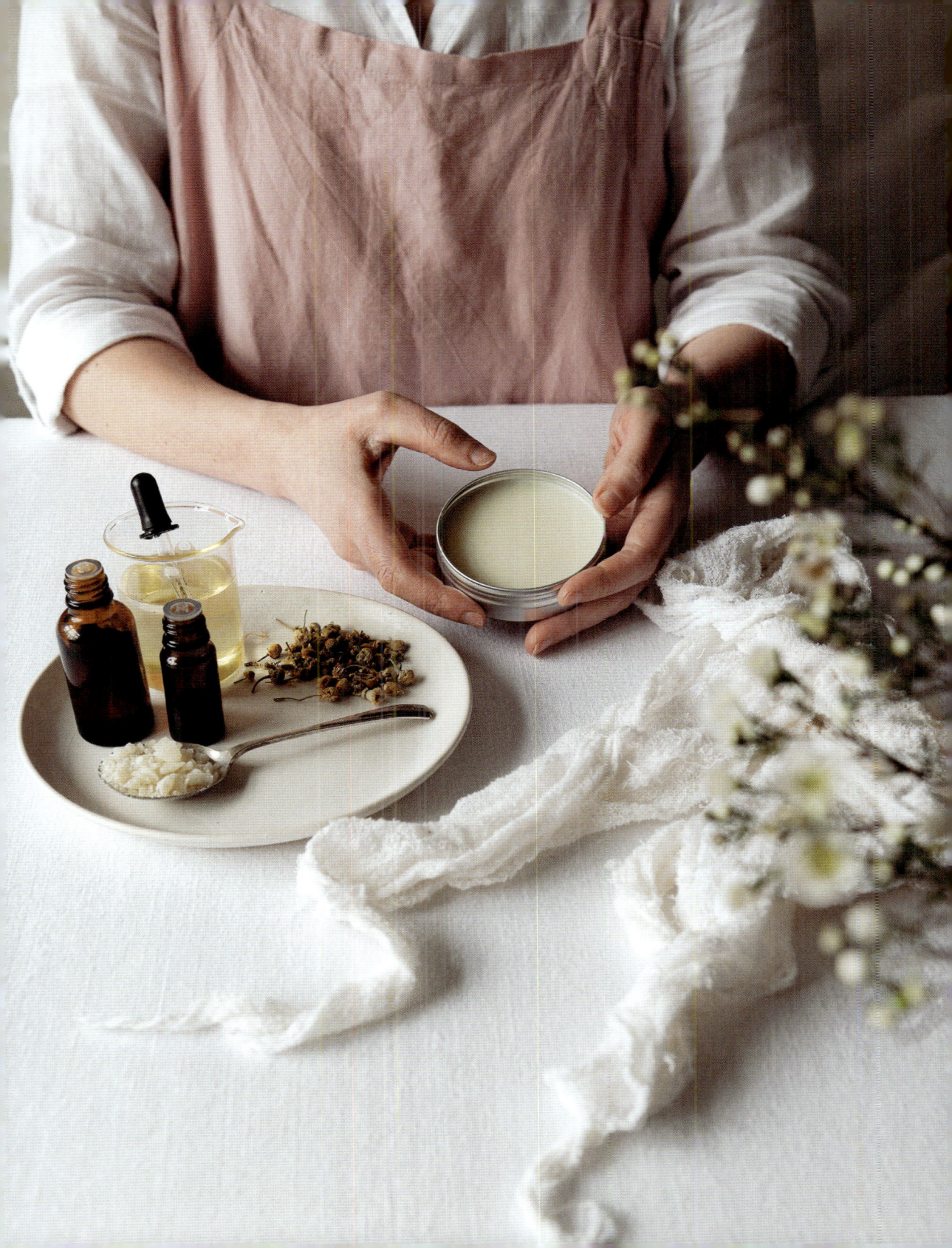

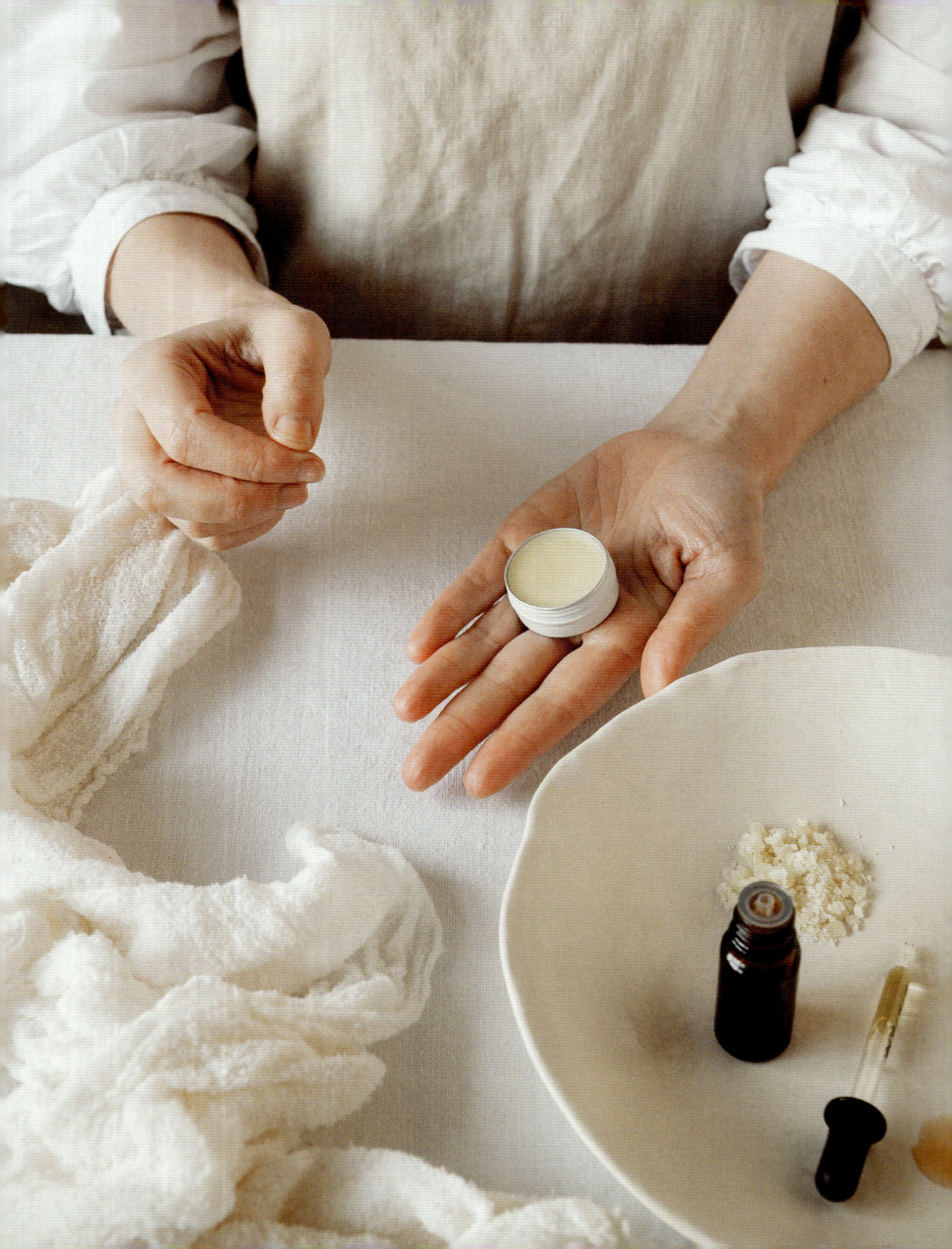

# HYDRATING LIP BALM

*I absolutely love a lip balm, and I still can't believe how easy they are to make! I make a batch of these quite regularly and gift them to my friends and family. These balms smell good enough to eat and are super soothing, too, and, of course, they are perfectly sized to travel with you wherever you go.*

Makes 4 small tins
(15 g [0.5 oz] each)

30 g (2 tbsp) sweet almond oil
15 g (1 tbsp) cocoa butter
10 g (3 tsp) beeswax
0.5 g vitamin E oil
0.5 g mandarin essential oil

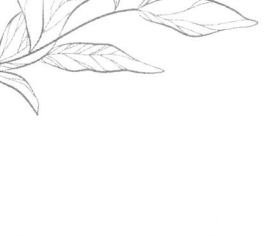

Using the double boiler method, gently melt the sweet almond oil, cocoa butter and beeswax until they are a liquid consistency. Read more about the double boiler method on page 146.

Take the mixture off the heat and place in the fridge. When the mixture has cooled to below 105°F (40°C), add the vitamin E oil and mandarin essential oil and stir to combine. This should take 10 to 15 minutes to cool.

Transfer to small containers and label.

## Get to Know Your Ingredients!

I just love to make a batch of these lip balms! They're so rich and nourishing and smell absolutely amazing; the blend of cocoa butter and mandarin essential oil is perfection. Adding beeswax to this balm is a perfect way to keep your lips hydrated, as the beeswax forms a protective barrier and protects the skin from moisture loss and harsh environmental factors, such as rough weather conditions and pollution.

# REPAIRING LIP BALM

*This is the perfect repairing lip butter to soothe your chapped lips and bring them back to life. It's a softer consistency to the lip balm recipe, and I like to massage a pea-sized amount into my lips before I fall asleep at night.*

*Makes* 4 small tins (15 g [0.5 oz] each)

20 g (1½ tbsp) apricot kernel oil
15 g (1 tbsp) mango butter
10 g (3 tsp) beeswax
10 g (3 tsp) castor oil
0.5 g vitamin E oil

Using the double boiler method, gently melt the apricot kernel oil, mango butter, beeswax and castor oil until they are a liquid consistency. Read more about using the double boiler method on page 146.

Take the mixture off the heat and place in the fridge. When it's cooled to below 105°F (40°C), add the vitamin E oil and stir to combine. This should take 10 to 15 minutes to cool.

Transfer to small containers and label. I like to use small tins, but I also find that 1-serving jam jars work really well, too, and are a great reuse!

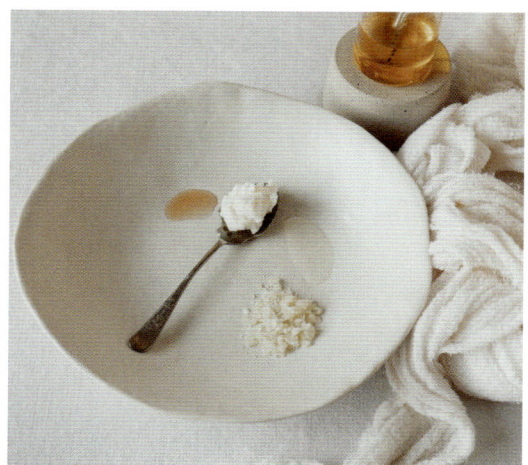

## Get to Know Your Ingredients!

I have included slow-penetrating oils in this recipe so that they take their time to nourish the outer layers of your skin while the beeswax forms a layer on the skin to protect it from further dryness. This is a deeply nourishing butter, and if you struggle with dry, chapped lips in winter, this will become your favorite product!

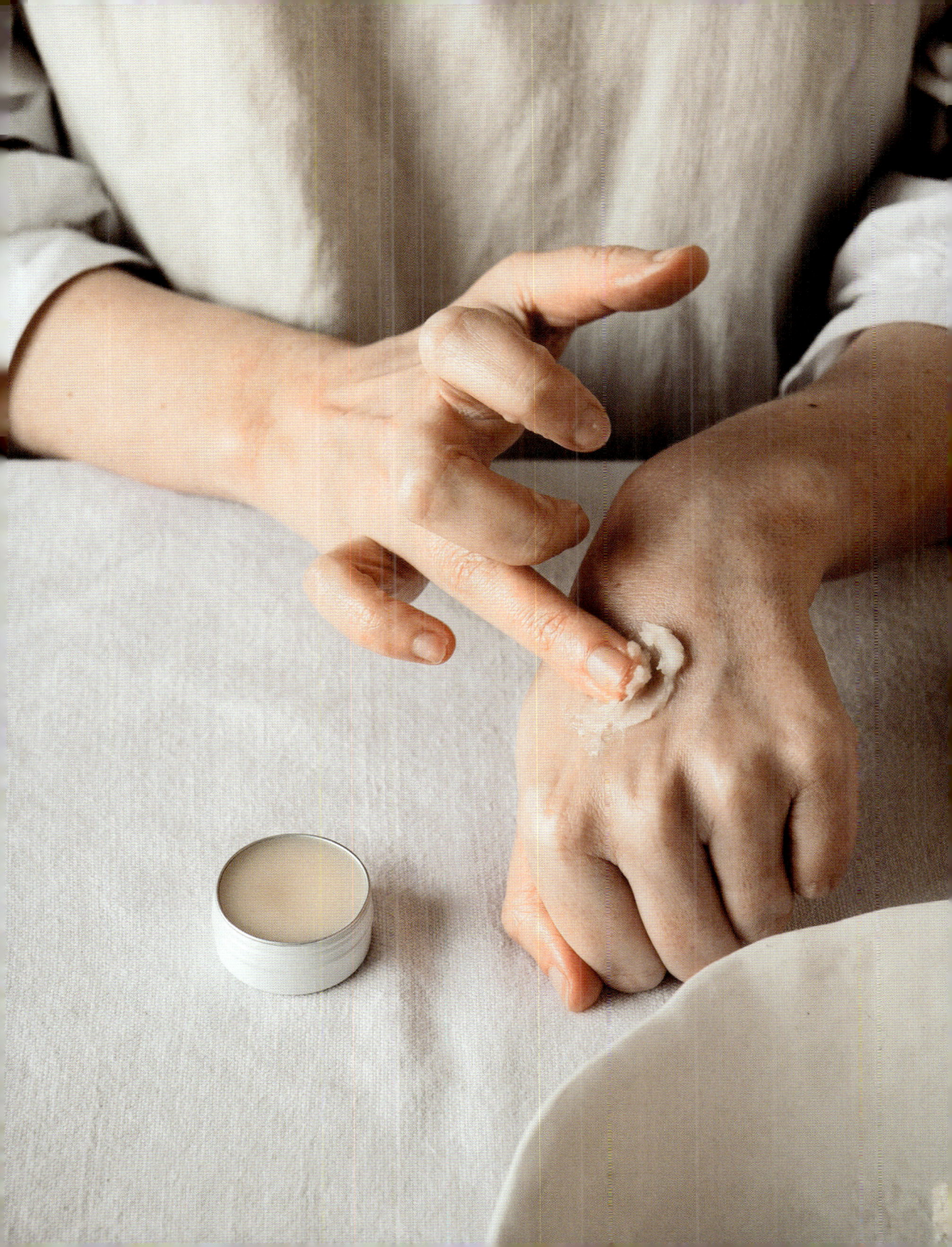

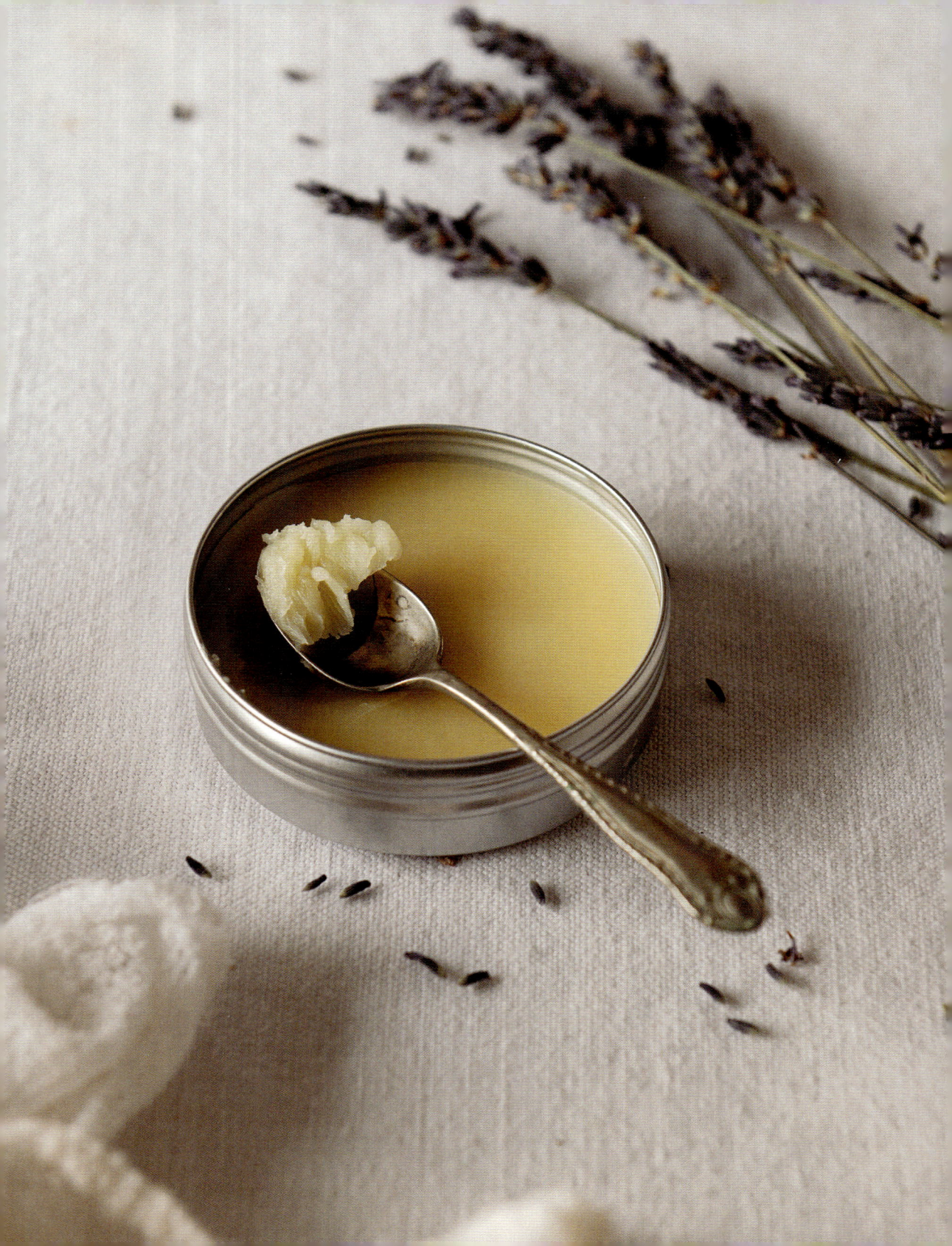

# AROMATHERAPY MASSAGE LOTION BALM

*This is a beautiful aromatherapy balm that is super easy to make. It is a softer consistency than the lotion bars and is easy to use. I recommend taking a generous amount, warming it up between the palm of your hands and massaging it deeply into your skin for as long as needed to help you relax and unwind.*

*Makes* 1 medium-sized jar (100 g [½ cup])

55 g (3½ tbsp) sweet almond oil
19 g (1½ tbsp) jojoba oil
15 g (1 tbsp) beeswax
10 g (3 tsp) mango butter
1 g vitamin E oil
0.6 g lavender essential oil
0.3 g geranium essential oil
0.1 g clove essential oil

Gently melt the sweet almond oil, jojoba oil, beeswax and mango butter using the double boiler method (read more about method on page 146).

When melted and blended together, take off the heat and allow to cool in the refrigerator. When mixture reaches below 77°F (25°C), add the vitamin E oil, lavender essential oil, geranium essential oil and clove essential oil. This should take 10 to 15 minutes to cool.

Add to a mold of your choice and place in the fridge overnight.

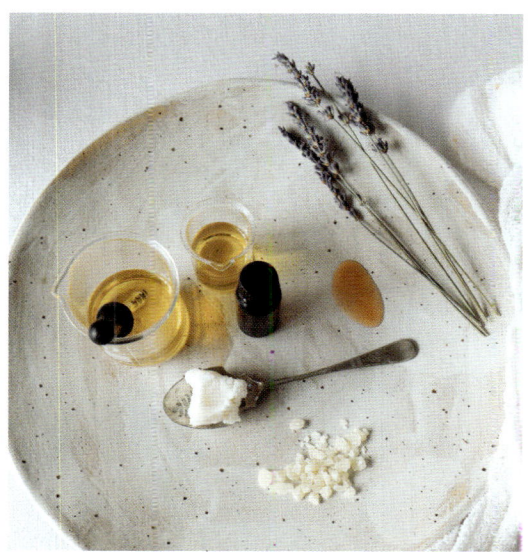

## Get to Know Your Ingredients!

As you warm up the lotion balm in your hands, breathe in the aroma that is released for extra relaxation. Lavender essential oil is naturally anti-bacterial, as well as helping to ease stress and aid sleeping, and clove essential oil is used aromatically to help alleviate pain and discomfort.

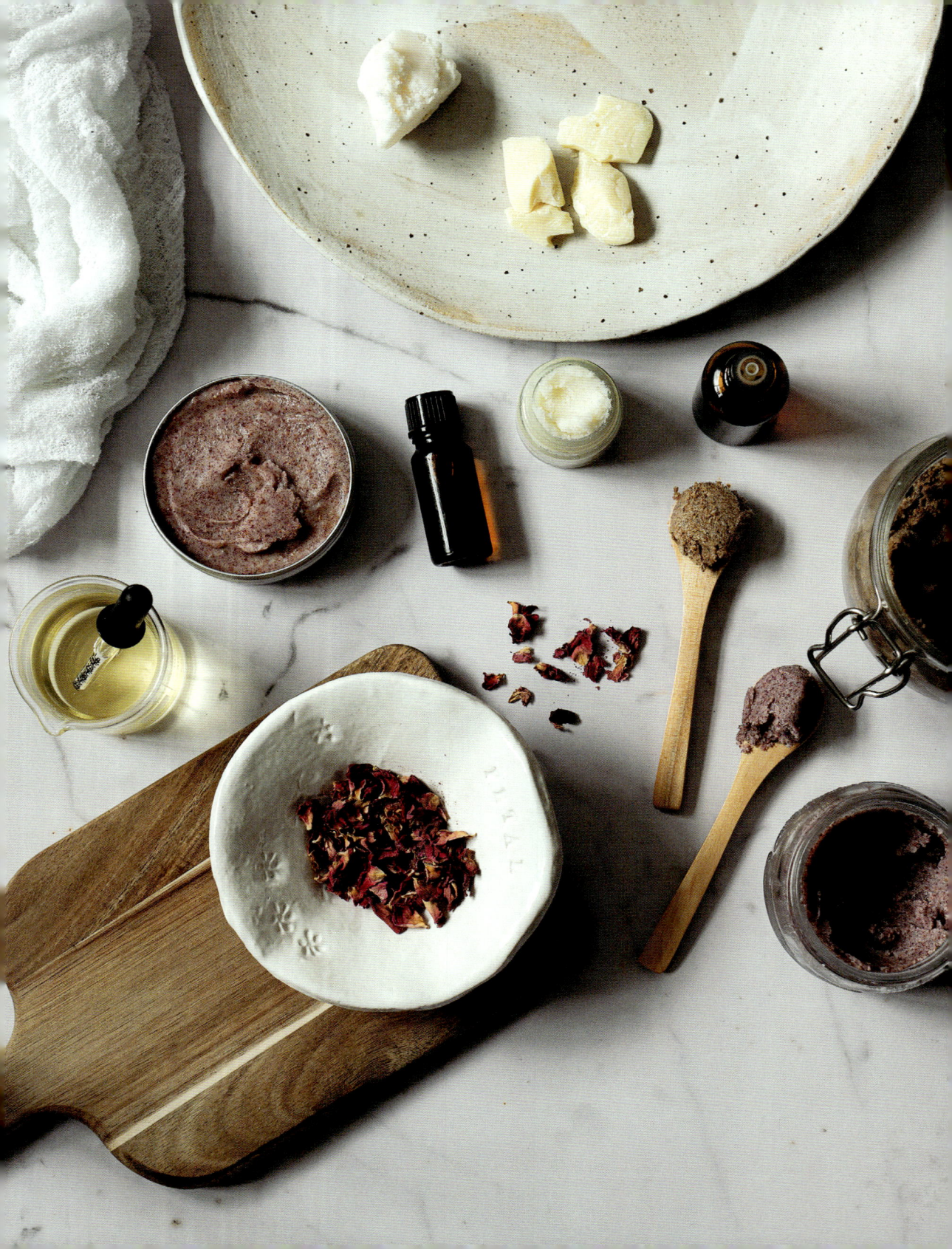

# SCRUBS

Face and body scrubs are the simplest thing to make on your kitchen table, and you can play around with them to make so many different varieties! I absolutely love to polish my skin with a good scrub once a week. It helps smooth my skin, encourages cell regeneration and allows all of our lovely lotions to be absorbed into the skin with ease.

You can use your scrubs in the bath or the shower. Simply start by wetting your skin thoroughly, then take a generous amount of the scrub and gently massage it into your skin using circular motions. Pay extra attention to areas where your skin needs extra love, like elbows, knees and heels.

You will notice that I have included preservatives in these recipes. Although these recipes are waterless, they are made to be used in the shower or bath, which could introduce water into the recipe. Therefore, we need to keep them safe for use.

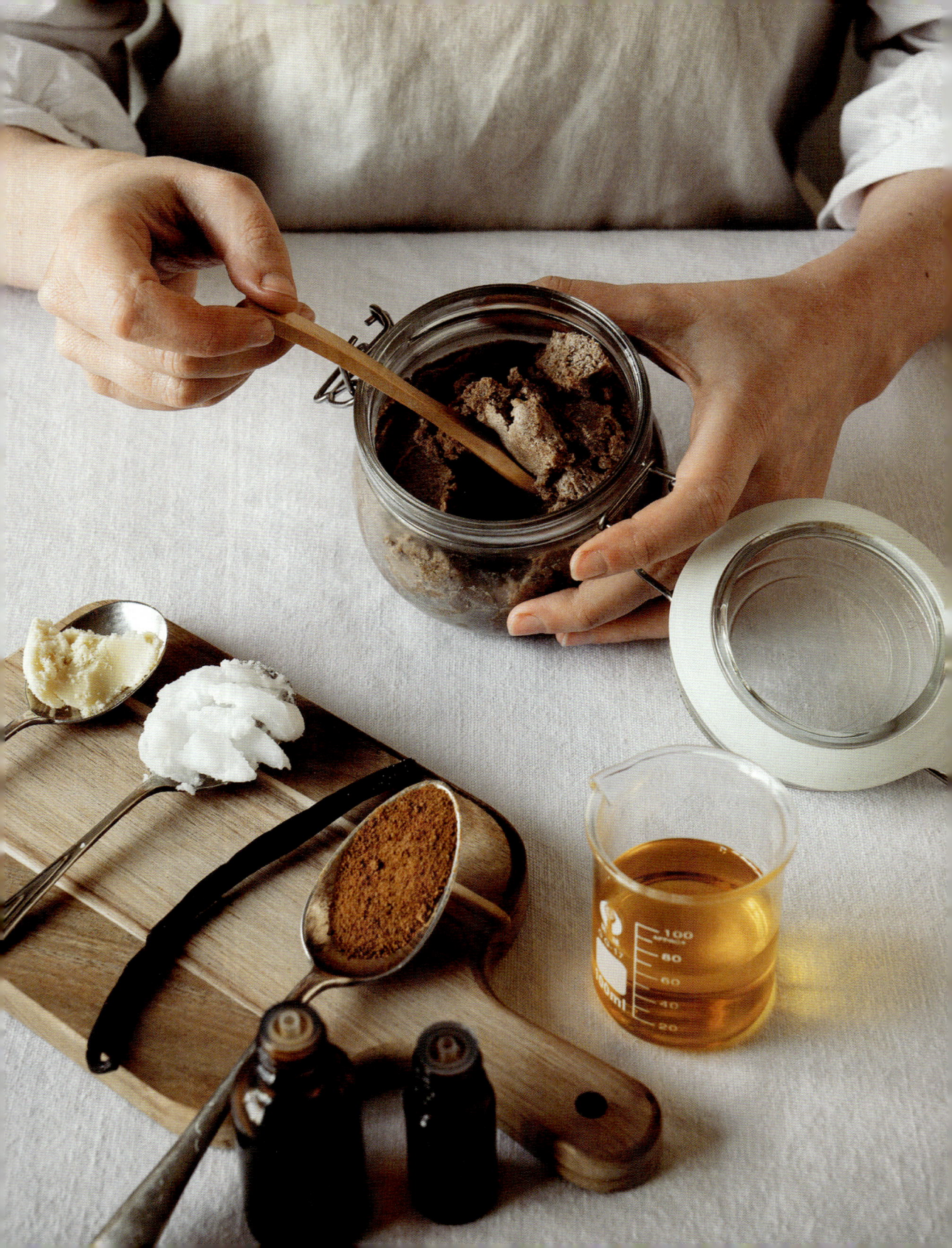

# INDULGENT SUGAR BODY SCRUB

*Your body will thank you for making this allover scrub. It's the perfect way to care for and nourish your skin and will give you a glow that lasts for days!*

*Makes* 1 medium-sized jar (100 g [½ cup])

55 g (3½ tbsp) coconut oil

30 g (2 tbsp) shea butter

80 g (½ cup) coconut sugar

21 g (1½ tbsp) Vanilla Pod Infused Oil (page 131)

20 g (1½ tbsp) sweet almond oil

2 g vitamin E oil

2 g preservative eco

1.5 g pure vanilla extract

0.5 g mandarin essential oil

In a large bowl, add the coconut oil and shea butter and gently melt using the double boiler method until liquid (read more about the double boiler method on page 146).

Place the liquid mixture in the fridge and allow to cool until it begins to solidify. This should take 30 to 60 minutes.

Add the coconut sugar and whisk using a handheld whisk until light and fluffy, which should take approximately 30 seconds.

Add the Vanilla Pod Infused Oil, sweet almond oil, vitamin E oil, preservative eco, pure vanilla extract and mandarin essential oil and return to the fridge until cool again. This should only take 3 to 5 minutes.

Whisk one more time and add to a clean, sterile container.

Scoop a generous handful and massage into damp skin whenever you find yourself needing pampering!

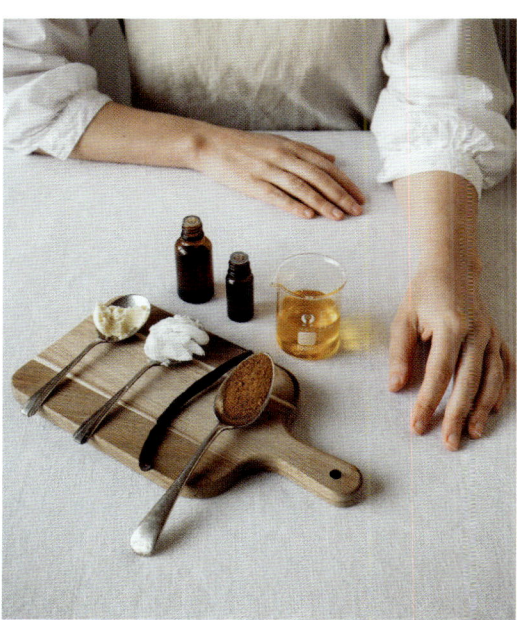

### Get to Know Your Ingredients!

I try to use this scrub once a week to exfoliate and encourage cell turnover. The coconut sugar in this recipe is gentle enough to exfoliate the skin without causing any damage. I have added shea butter and coconut oil to this recipe, which are nourishing and deeply moisturizing for your skin.

# GLOWING FACE POLISH

*I love to use this rose petal infused face scrub once a week to remove dead skin cells and soften my skin. Using a scrub weekly also helps to improve your skin tone and texture.*

---

*Makes* 1 medium-sized jar (100 g [½ cup])

---

35 g (2 tbsp) coconut oil

15 g (1½ tbsp) rosehip oil

13 g (3 tsp) mango butter

30 g (¼ cup) caster sugar

4 g (1 tsp) ground rose petals

1 g vitamin E oil

1 g preservative eco

0.5 g geranium essential oil

0.5 g lavender essential oil

In a large bowl, add the coconut oil, rosehip oil and mango butter and gently melt using the double boiler method until liquid. Read more about the double boiler method on page 146.

Place the liquid mixture in the fridge and allow to cool until it begins to solidify. This should take approximately 1 hour.

Add the caster sugar and ground rose petals, then whisk until light and fluffy.

Add the vitamin E oil, preservative eco, geranium essential oil and lavender essential oil and return to the fridge for a few minutes to cool. Whisk again for approximately 30 seconds and transfer to a clean, sterile container.

Use weekly as an exfoliating face polish.

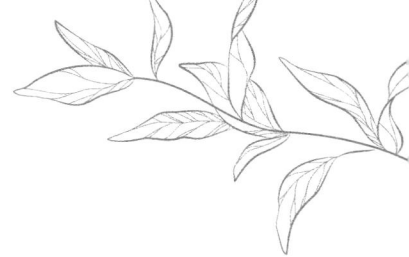

## Get to Know Your Ingredients!

When making a scrub for the face, it's really important to use ingredients that are gentle enough for delicate skin. Caster sugar scrubs are a great alternative to more abrasive scrubs that have large granules or hard particles and can help reveal a brighter complexion by gently buffing away those dead skin cells.

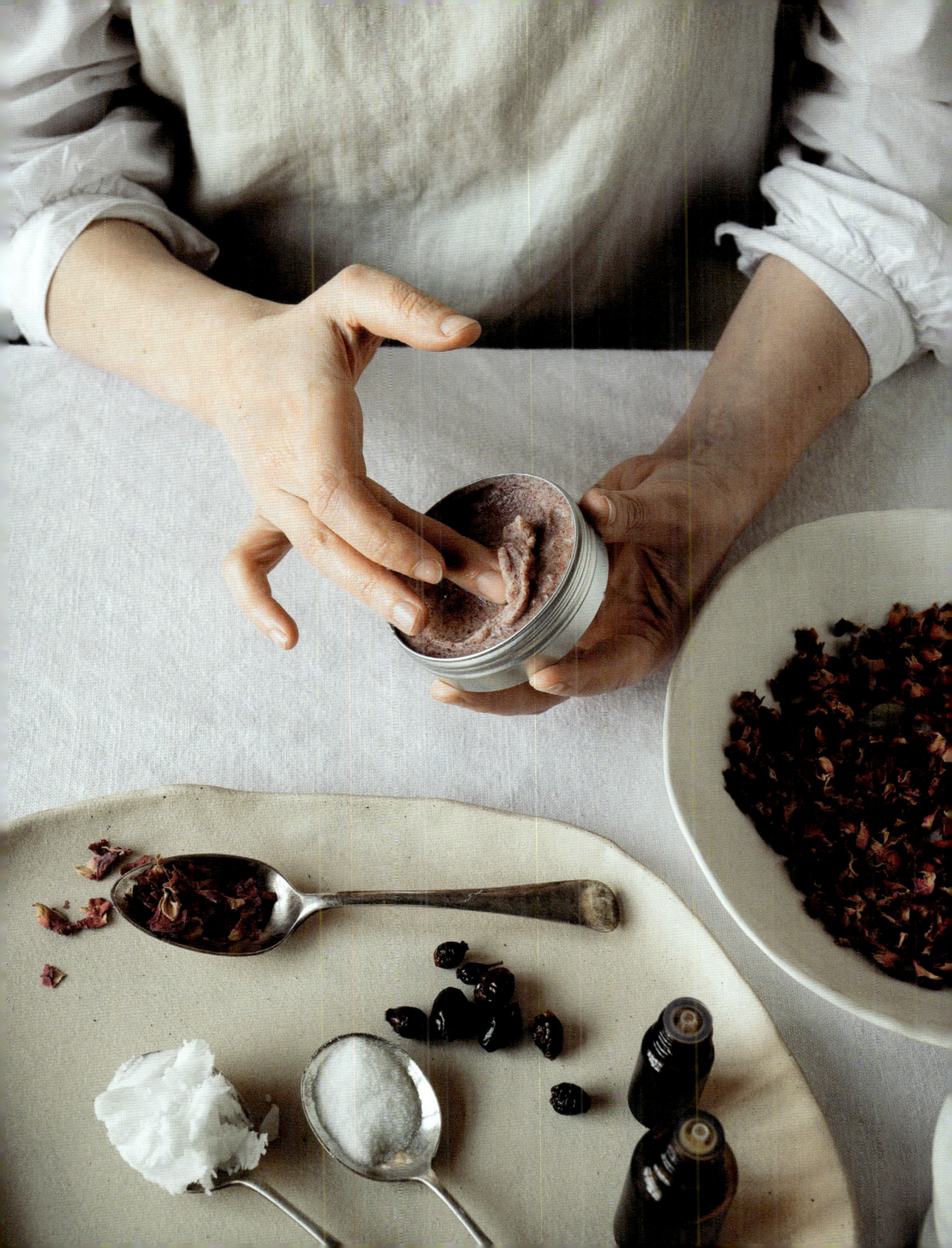

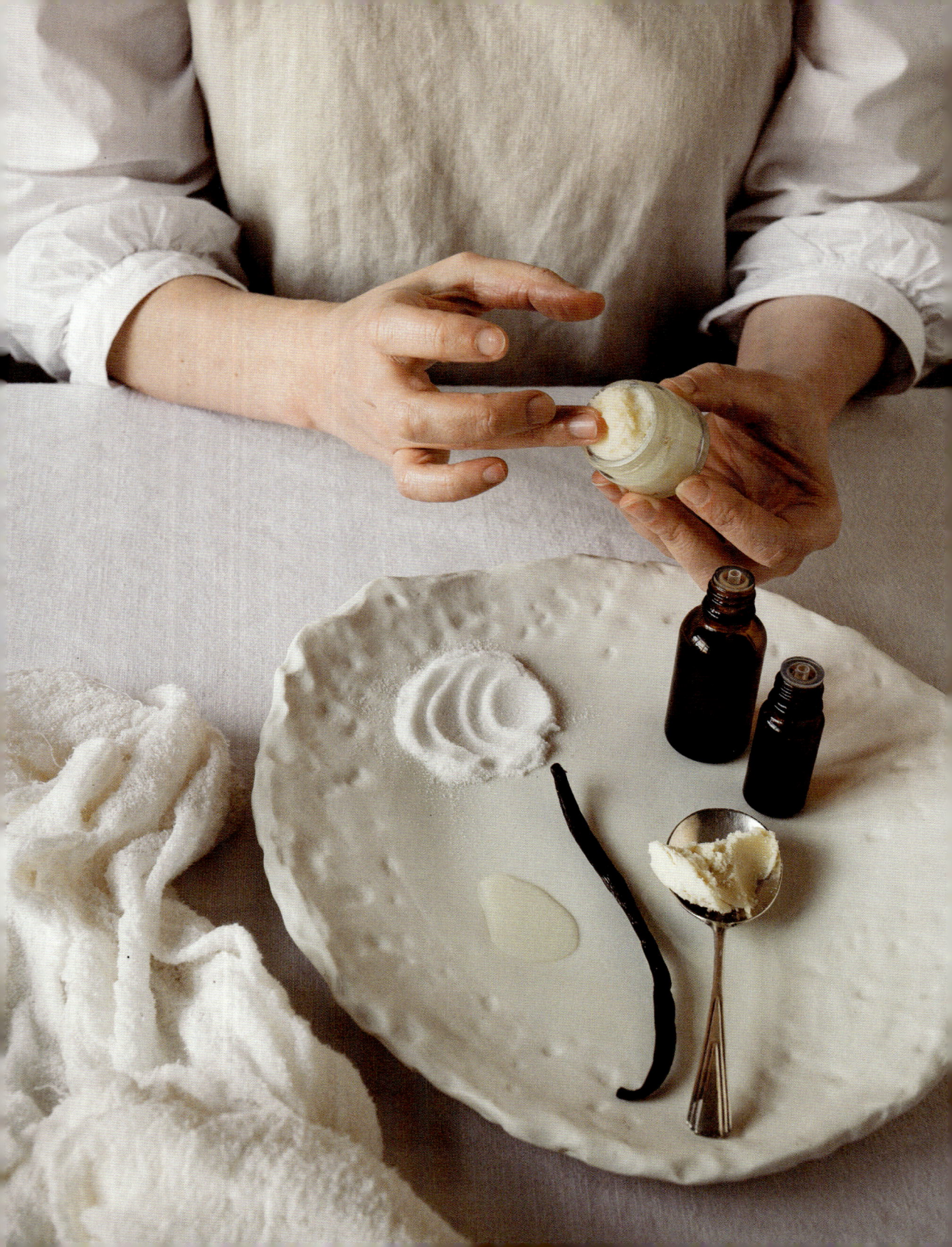

# PLUMPING PEPPERMINT AND VANILLA LIP SCRUB

*Similarly to the face, your lips need pampering too—particularly in the harsh weather! The skin on the lips is thinner and more delicate than the skin on the rest of your face, which makes it more susceptible to dryness and damage. This little jar of scrub is the ultimate skin-smoothing scrub for your lips. The butters and oils help to protect your lips while the sugar helps to buff away any dead skin.*

*Makes* 1 small jar (50 g [⅛ cup])

11 g (3 tsp) shea butter

6 g (1 tsp) castor oil

6 g (1 tsp) Vanilla Pod Infused Oil (page 131)

25 g (¼ cup) caster sugar

0.7 g vanilla essence

0.5 g vitamin E oil

0.5 g preservative eco

0.3 g peppermint essential oil

In a bowl, add the shea butter, castor oil and Vanilla Pod Infused Oil and gently melt using the double boiler method until liquid. Read more about the double boiler method on page 146.

Place the liquid mixture in the fridge and allow to cool until it begins to solidify. This should take approximately 30 minutes.

Add the caster sugar and whisk until light and fluffy.

Add the vanilla essence, vitamin E oil, preservative eco and peppermint essential oil and return to the fridge for a few minutes to cool. Whisk again for approximately 30 seconds and transfer to a clean, sterile container.

Use whenever you feel your lips need a little TLC.

## Get to Know Your Ingredients!

This lip scrub is gentle enough to use on the lips while the castor oil is deeply moisturizing. The small granules of caster sugar in this recipe allows for natural exfoliation and helps topical products be applied easily. Follow up with Repairing Lip Balm (page 62) for the ultimate lip treatment.

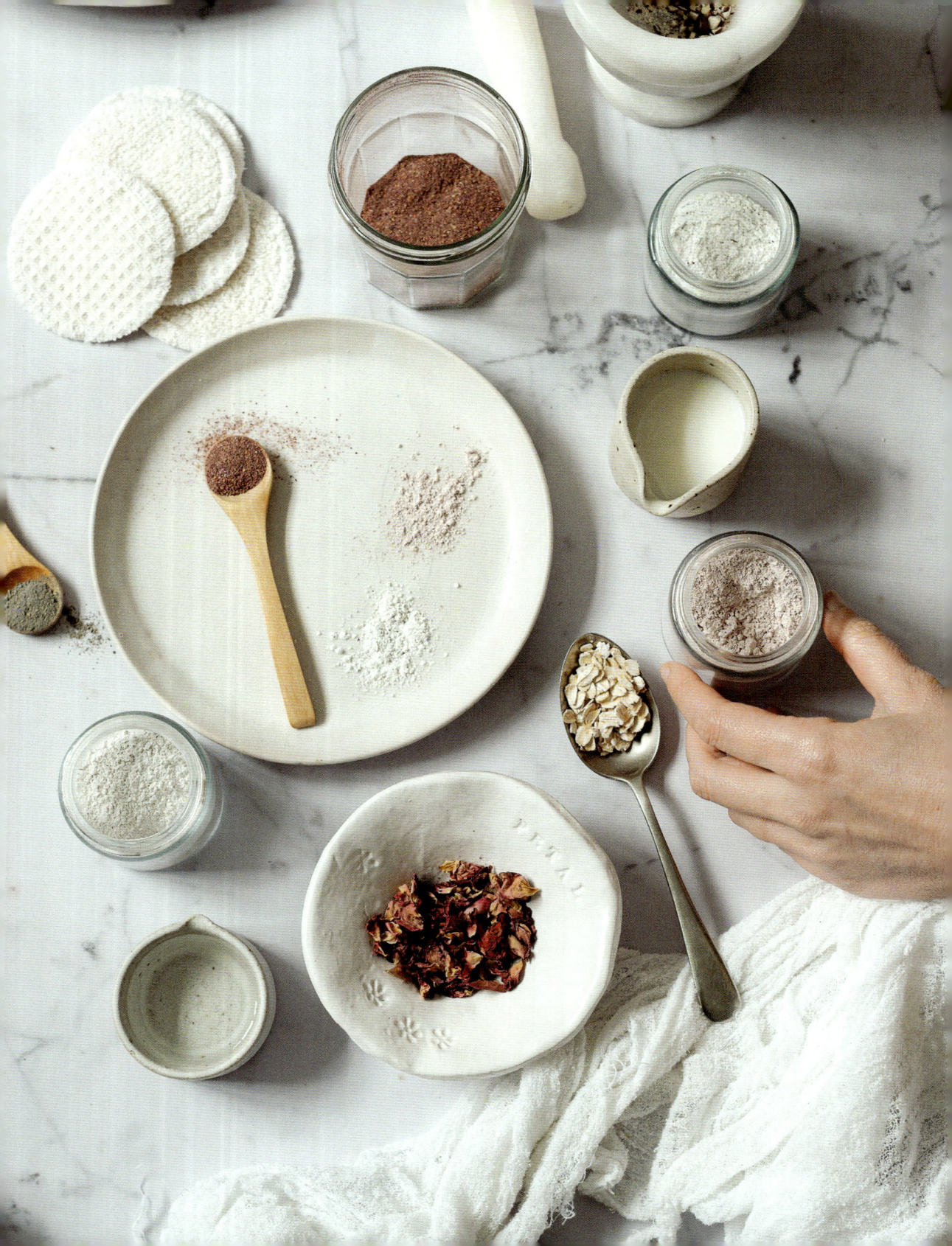

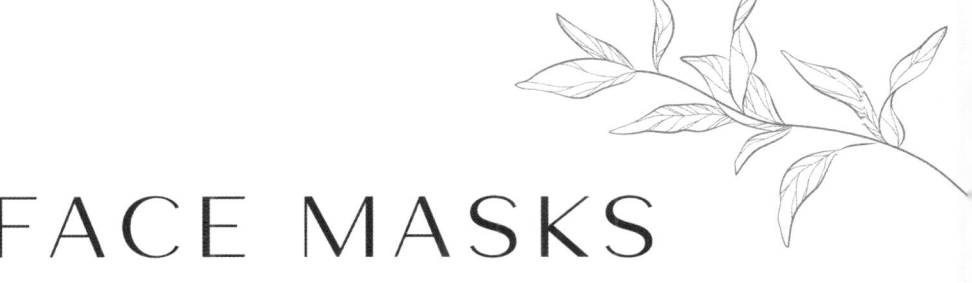

# FACE MASKS

I am showcasing some beautiful clays that you can use as face masks in this chapter of the book. I love how they are so low maintenance yet so effective in deeply cleansing the skin. Face masks should be used on clean skin and only need to be used weekly to help smooth, soften and cleanse.

I have chosen to create these clay recipes as "two-part" recipes for a number of reasons. Firstly, when clay is introduced to water of any kind, it becomes very difficult to preserve, so it's safer to keep it separate. Secondly, you can add lots of different "liquids" to your clay masks to make them different every time! Finally, your masks will last so much longer by creating them this way. There is no risk of them spoiling, and they store really easily in your bathroom cabinet.

When you choose to use your masks, you can add the clay powder to a liquid to create them. The powder should make up to ten face masks.

It is entirely your choice which liquid you choose to add to the mask. Water is a great addition to activate all of the minerals in the clay, but you can also choose to add a hydrosol, milk or even honey, which have additional skin-loving properties.

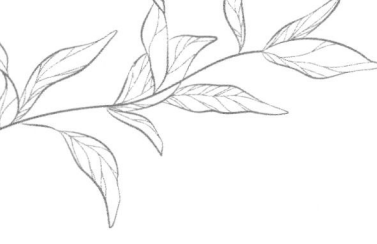

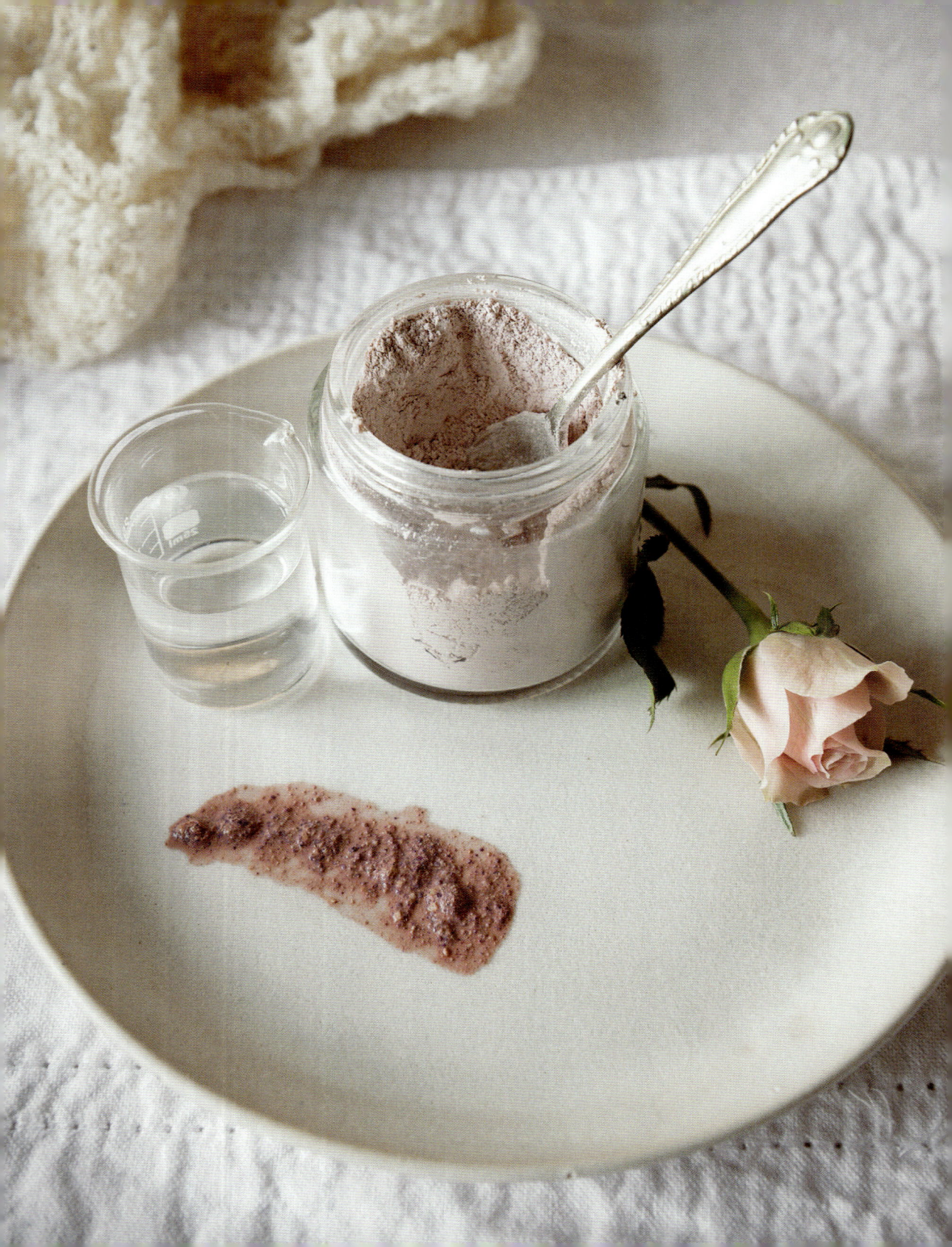

# ROSE CLAY HYDRATING FACE MASK

*This is a beautiful mask that is gentle yet deeply cleansing at the same time. It is great for combination skin types and gentle enough to be used weekly to help reset your skin and bring a lovely glow to your face*

*Makes* 1 small jar (50 g [⅛ cup])

5 g (½ tbsp) rose petals
45 g (2 cups) rose kaolin clay

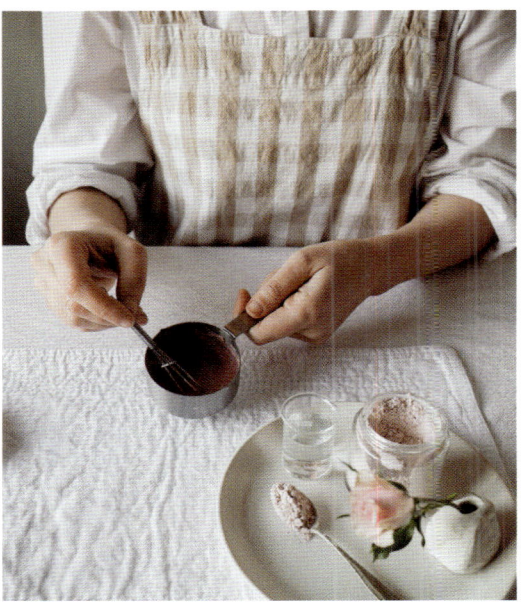

Using a pestle and mortar or an electric grinder, grind your rose petals so that they become a very fine powder.

Place the rose kaolin clay in a bowl and add the petal powder.

Transfer to a clean, sterile jar until ready to use.

To activate the mask, take a tablespoon (15 g) of the dry clay mixture using a clean, dry spoon and add 2 tablespoons of liquid (30 ml) and mix. You can use water, hydrosol, milk or honey as the liquid.

Apply a thin layer to clean, damp skin. Leave until the clay dries and then wipe away with a warm face cloth.

This is a product that needs to be stored separately until you choose to use it. The powder should make up to ten masks.

## Get to Know Your Ingredients!

Rose kaolin clay is a balancing clay that helps to address both oily and dry areas of skin. It is a mild clay and suitable for sensitive or dry skin types. Combined with powdered rose petals, this clay mask provides gentle cleansing and helps to remove dirt and excess oils.

Each of these masks will provide numerous benefits when mixed with water.

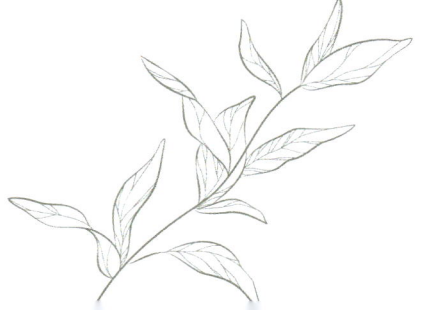

# GREEN CLAY DEEP CLEANSE FACE MASK

*This mask is a hero for oily skin types. It is super cleansing and contains numerous minerals. It is a mask that can be used weekly on acne-prone and oily skin but may be less suitable to use this often for sensitive skin types.*

Makes 1 small jar (50 g [⅛ cup])

5 g (½ tbsp) chamomile
45 g (2 cups) green clay

Using a pestle and mortar or an electric grinder, grind your chamomile until it resembles a fine powder.

In a small bowl, mix together the chamomile powder and green clay and store in a clean, sterile container.

To activate the mask, take a tablespoon (15 g) of the dry clay mixture using a clean, dry spoon and add 2 tablespoons of liquid (30 ml) and mix. You can use water, hydrosol, milk or honey as the liquid.

Cleanse the skin using a cleanser of your choice and apply this mask to damp skin. Leave until the clay dries and then wipe away with a warm face cloth.

This is a product that needs to be stored separately until you choose to use it. The powder should make up to ten masks.

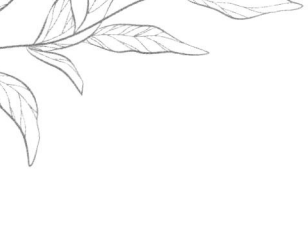

## Get to Know Your Ingredients!

Green clay contains up to ten mineral oxides, including magnesium, calcium, potassium, dolomite, silica, manganese, phosphorus, silicon, copper and selenium. It is one of the most detoxifying ingredients that you can use on your skin. It helps remove impurities from the skin and can also improve the tone and texture of your skin.

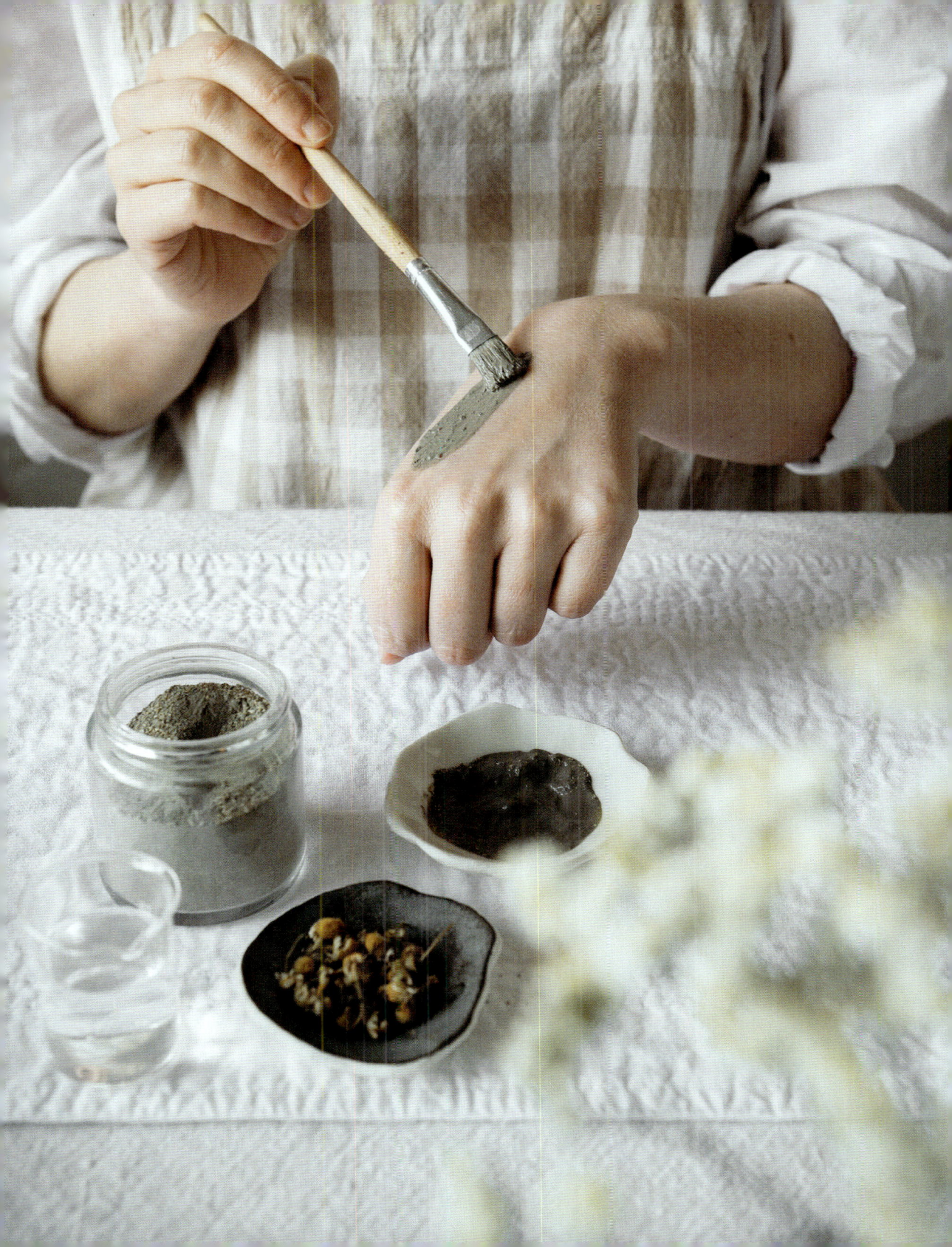

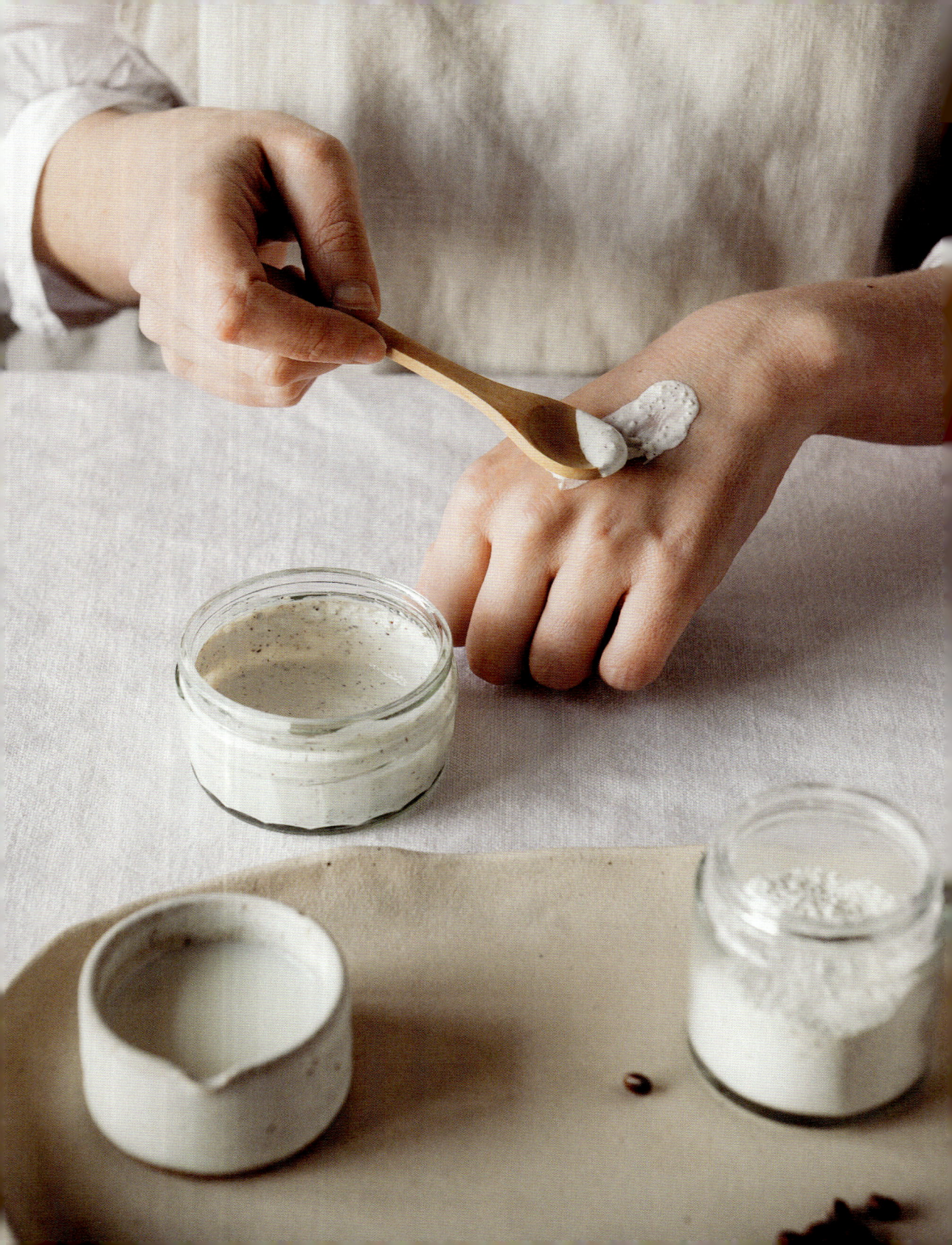

# KAOLIN CARING CLAY MASK

*This is created using white kaolin clay and ground adzuki beans. If you enjoy making the Deep Muscle Massaging Bar (page 49) using adzuki beans, you will find that you can also use the adzuki beans for this recipe. I love creating products where ingredients have a crossover. It's a great way to learn how ingredients can be multipurpose. This is another mask that is suitable for normal and sensitive skin types. Make sure that the adzuki beans are finely ground so that they provide a gentle exfoliation.*

*Makes* 1 small jar (50 g [⅛ cup])

10 g (1 tbsp) adzuki beans
40 g (2 cups) white kaolin clay

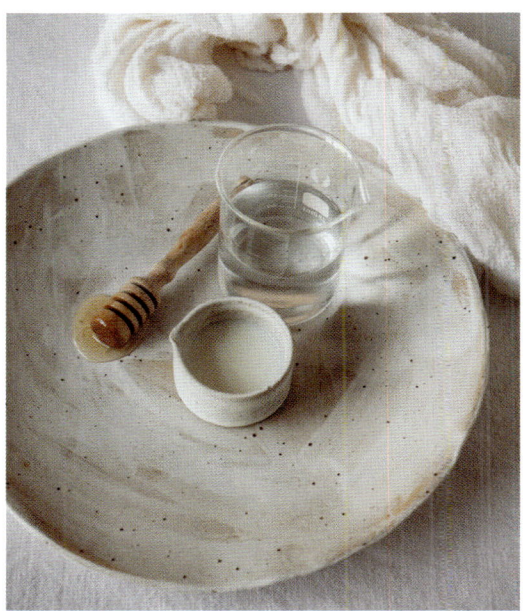

Using a pestle and mortar or an electric grinder, grind your adzuki beans until they resemble a powder. Mix together the ground adzuki beans and white kaolin clay and store in a clean, sterile container.

To activate the mask, take a tablespoon (15 g) of the dry clay mixture using a clean, dry spoon and add 2 tablespoons of liquid (30 ml) and mix. You can use water, hydrosol, milk or honey as the liquid.

Apply a thin layer to clean, damp skin. Leave until the clay dries and then wipe away with a warm face cloth.

This is a product that needs to be stored separately until you choose to use it. The powder should make up to ten masks.

## Get to Know Your Ingredients!

The kaolin clay in this recipe helps to remove dirt and excess oil, and gives a velvety feel to the skin. It also contains high levels of silica, which can help with skin rejuvenation. Adzuki beans contain saponins and are naturally cleansing, as well as being gently exfoliating. They also have absorbent properties, making them a great addition to use to help control excess oil on the skin.

# CALMING OAT FACE MASK

*This is the gentlest mask that I have included in these recipes and is suitable for the most sensitive skin types. It is still deeply cleansing and will leave your skin feeling soft and soothed with a beautiful glow. Apply weekly for great results.*

*Makes* 1 small jar (50 g [⅛ cup])

10 g (2 tbsp) oats
40 g (2 cups) kaolin clay

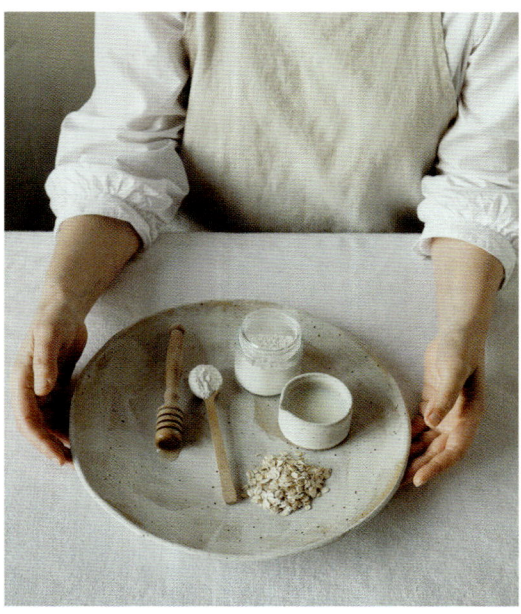

Using a pestle and mortar or an electric grinder, grind your oats until they resemble a powder. Mix together the oat powder and kaolin clay and store in a clean, sterile container.

To activate the mask, take a tablespoon (10 g) of the dry clay mixture and add approximately 1 teaspoon of liquid and mix using a spatula. You can use hydrosol, water, milk or honey as the liquid.

Cleanse the skin using a cleanser of your choice and apply this mask to damp skin. Leave until the clay dries and then wipe away with a warm muslin cloth.

This is a product that needs to be stored separately until you choose to use it. The powder should make three to four masks.

## Get to Know Your Ingredients!

This face mask is for the most sensitive skin. Kaolin clay has a soothing effect on the skin and can help to reduce inflammation and calm irritated skin. The finely ground oats contain antioxidants and help to relieve discomfort associated with dry skin conditions. The fine oat powder also provides gentle exfoliation and helps to remove dead skin cells without causing irritation.

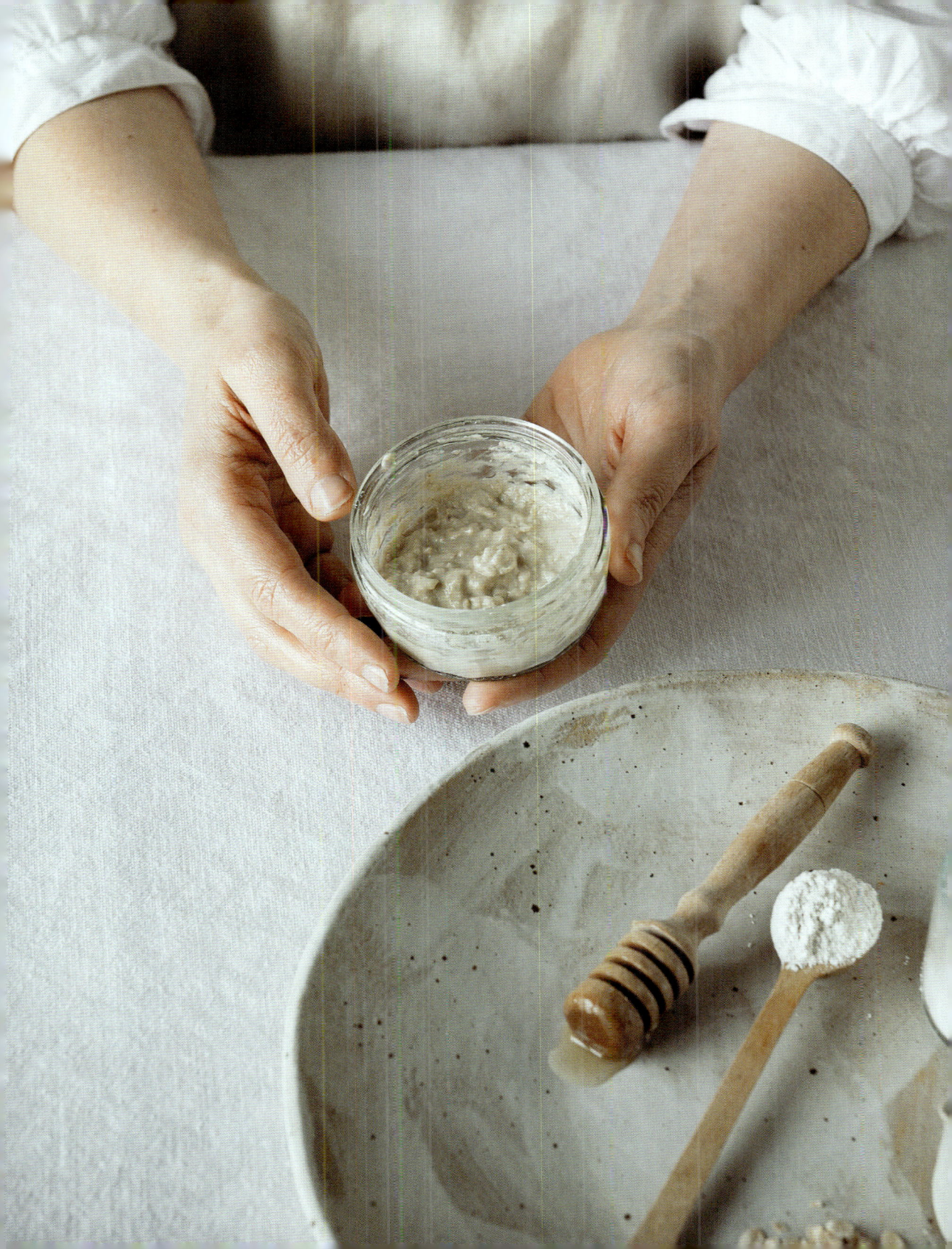

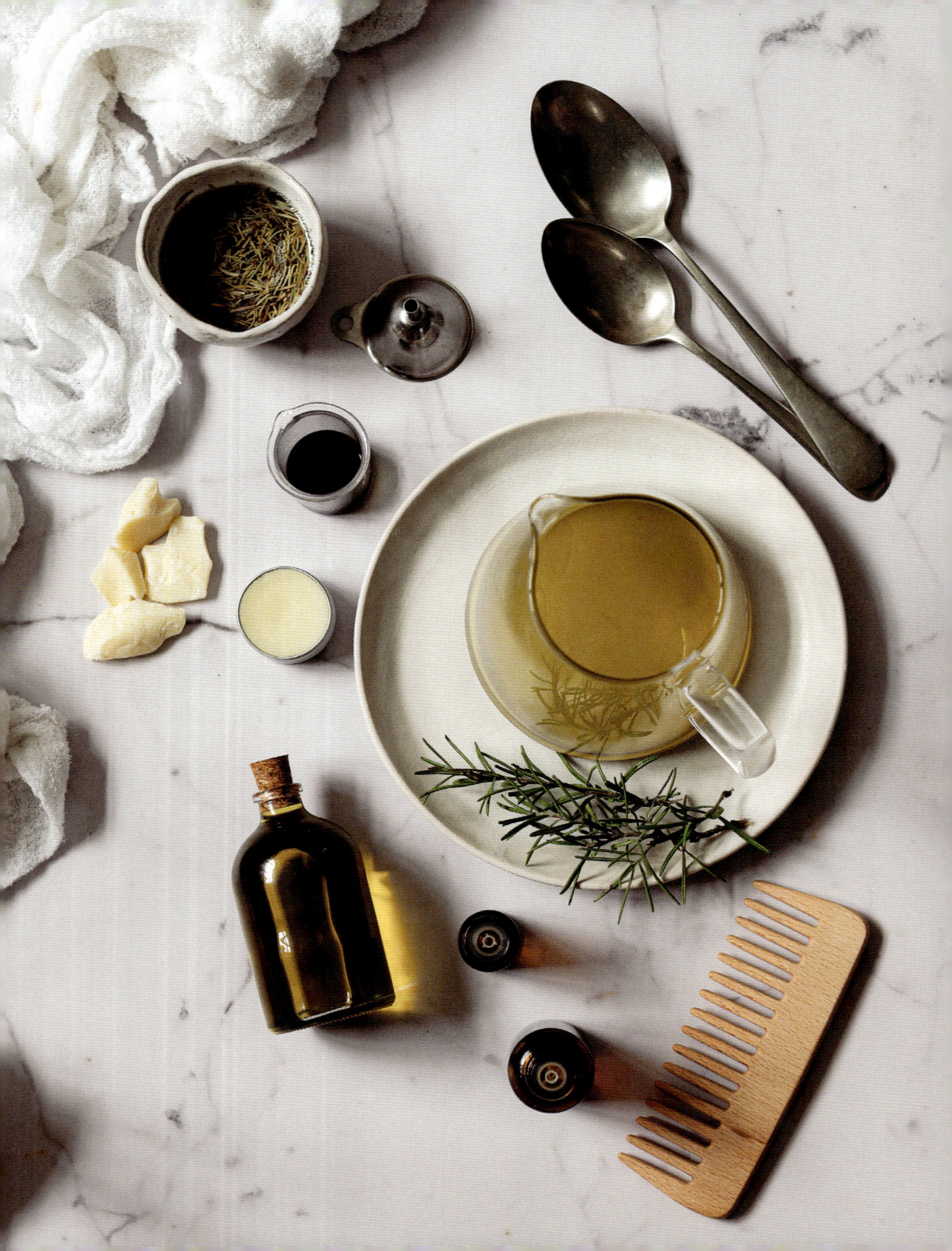

# TREATMENT OILS

I am sharing some of my favorite oil blends to showcase how effective they are for soothing and restoring the skin and hair. It always stuns me how much these products cost to buy at stores when they can be made so simply at home, with much better and more powerful ingredients.

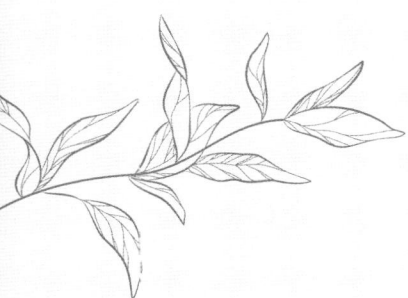

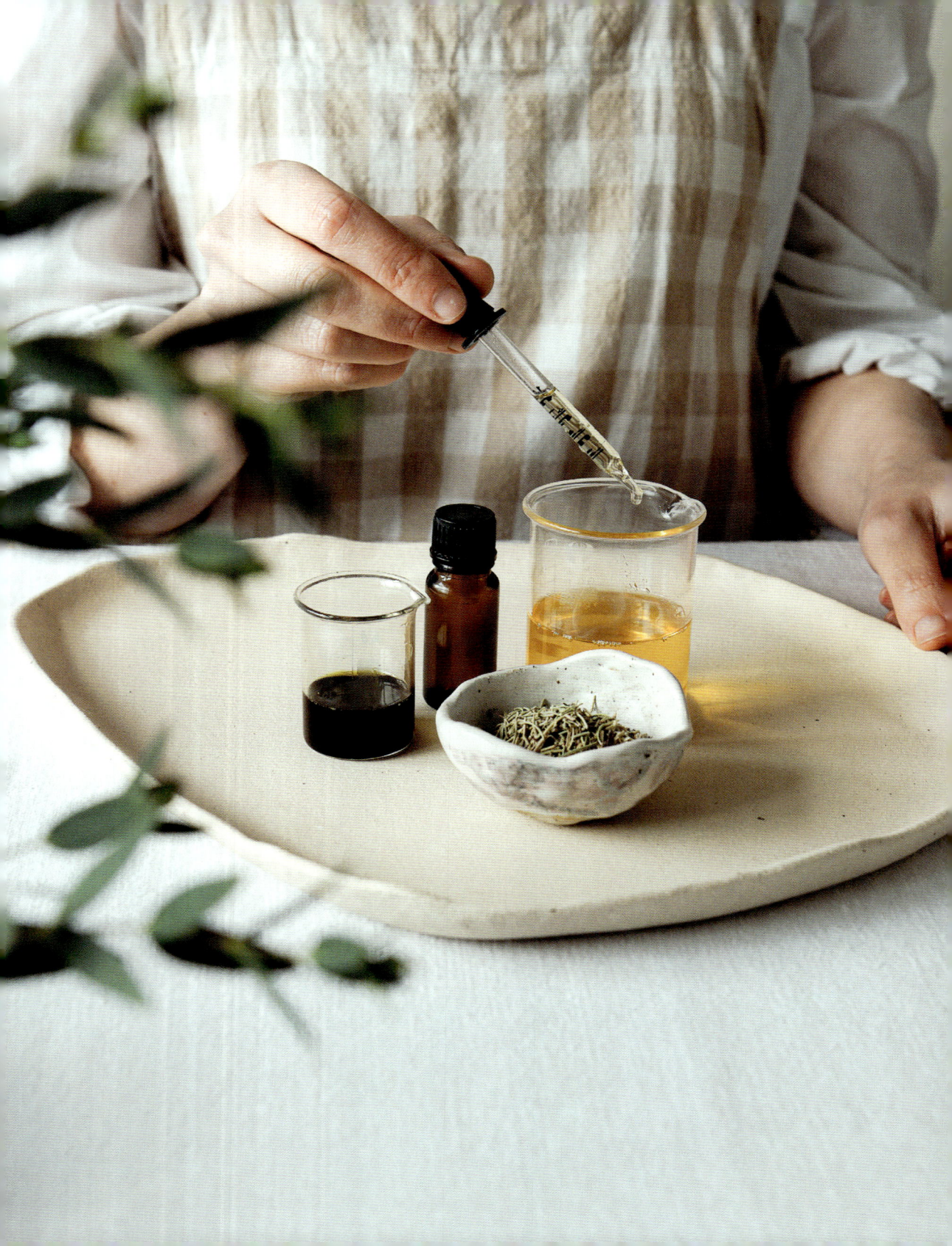

# HAIR GROWTH OIL

*The ingredients that I have included in this recipe all combine to really nourish your hair and encourage hair growth. I lost so much hair after having my children and found that even the texture of my hair changed and became very dry and weak. After using this treatment on my hair, it has returned to its previous health—shiny and nourished!*

*Makes* 1 medium-sized bottle (100 ml [⅓ cup])

49 g (3 tbsp) castor oil

30 g (2 tbsp) Rosemary Infused Oil (page 123)

20 g (1½ tbsp) hemp seed oil

0.5 g rosemary essential oil

0.5 g peppermint essential oil

In a bowl, combine the castor oil, Rosemary Infused Oil, hemp seed oil, rosemary essential oil and peppermint essential oil. Transfer to a medium-sized sterile bottle. I like to use a pipette dropper so that I can dispense a few drops onto my scalp.

Massage into the scalp and leave for at least 30 minutes before washing your hair. I like to leave it overnight so that the oils nourish and condition my scalp and strengthen my hair.

When you have used this treatment, it is advisable to shampoo your hair twice before conditioning. This is advisable as your daily shampoo and condition routine, but many people skip the second shampoo.

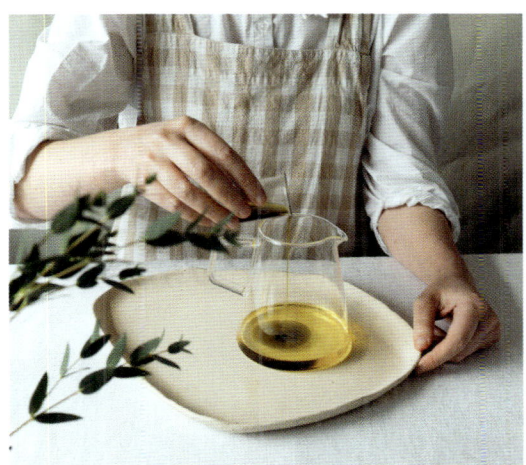

## Get to Know Your Ingredients!

Castor oil has been used for many years in hair care. It contains ricinoleic acid, which has been reported to help stimulate hair growth, contributing to thicker, longer hair. Rosemary has also been linked to promoting hair growth by improving blood circulation to the scalp. These two ingredients are like a "superfood" for maintaining healthy, strong hair. Peppermint essential oil has antimicrobial properties that can help soothe your scalp, while the cooling sensation can also help promote blood circulation.

# SOOTHE YOUR SKIN MASSAGE OIL

*Just writing this recipe was like a good massage! Did you know how many benefits there are to massages? Mood enhancement, stress reduction, improved sleep, immune system support—the list of benefits is lengthy! I used to limit massages and only have them as a treat because the massage oils available in the store were always so expensive. This is why I have created a massage oil that is both effective and really affordable.*

*Makes* 1 medium-sized bottle (100 ml [⅓ cup])

40 g (2½ tbsp) olive oil

30 g (2 tbsp) sweet almond oil

10 g (3 tsp) castor oil

10 g (3 tsp) Vanilla Pod Infused Oil (page 131)

7 g (3 tsp) Lavender Infused Oil (page 119)

1.5 g vitamin E oil

1 g lavender essential oil

0.3 g geranium essential oil

0.2 g rosemary essential oil

In a bowl, combine the olive oil, sweet almond oil, castor oil, Vanilla Pod Infused Oil, Lavender Infused Oil, vitamin E oil, lavender essential oil, geranium essential oil and rosemary essential oil.

Transfer to a small sterile bottle. When using, apply a good tablespoon (15 ml) of oil to the palm of your hand and rub your palms together to release the blend of essential oils. Take the time to massage into your skin for deep relaxation.

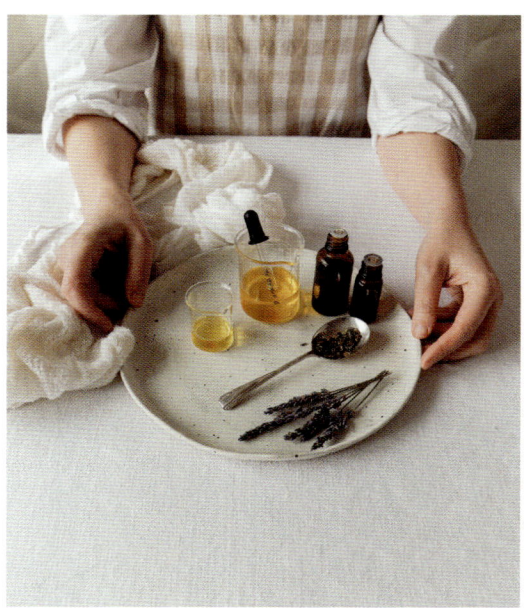

## Get to Know Your Ingredients!

A massage oil shouldn't penetrate the skin too quickly, which is why I have created this beautiful blend of oils using olive oil and castor oil. Olive oil is a great oil for massaging as it has a medium-slow penetration. It is also an effective moisturizer that helps to hydrate and soften the skin. The addition of the essential oils, Vanilla Pod Infused Oil and Lavender Infused Oil makes this massage oil wonderfully calming and helps relieve stress and uplift your mood.

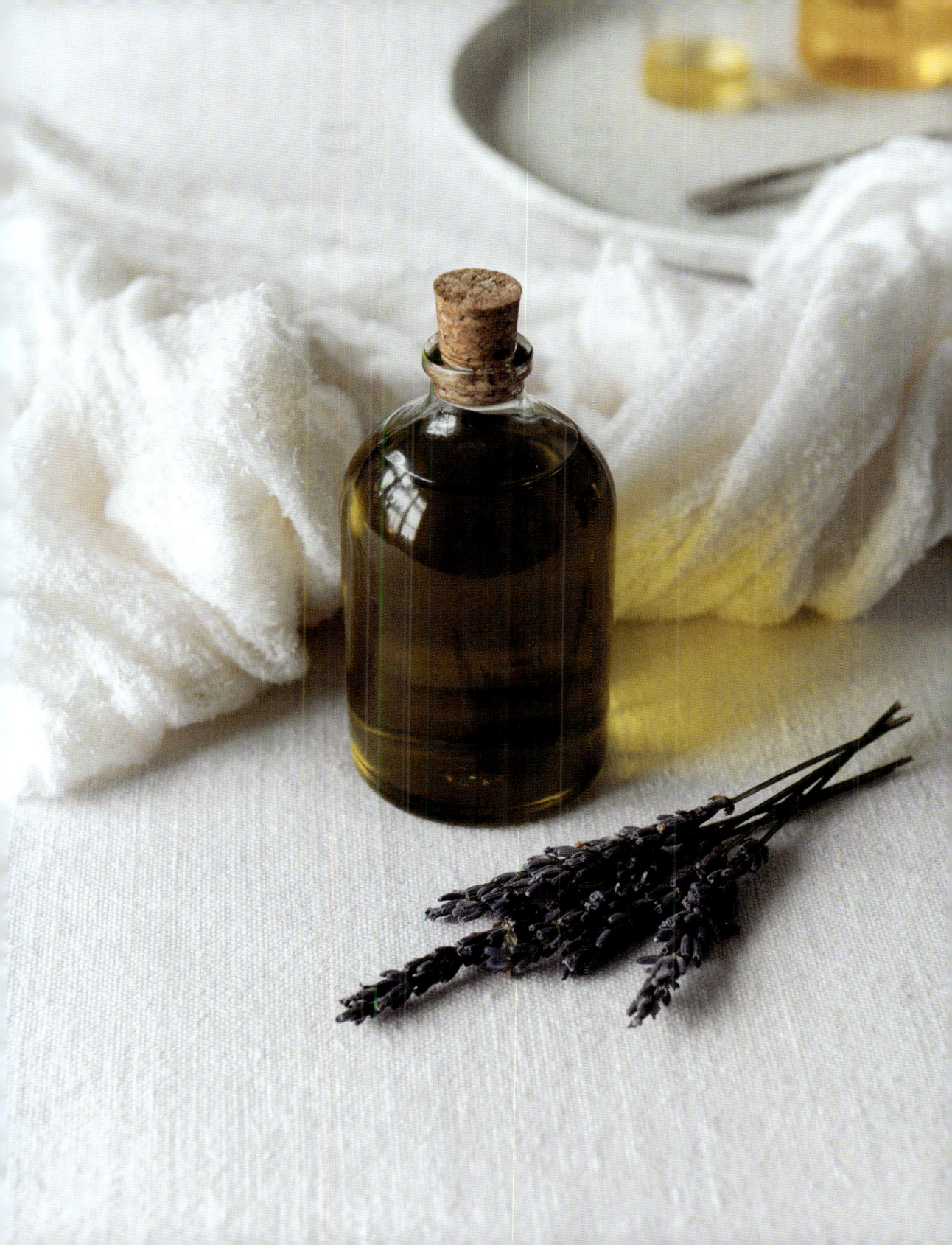

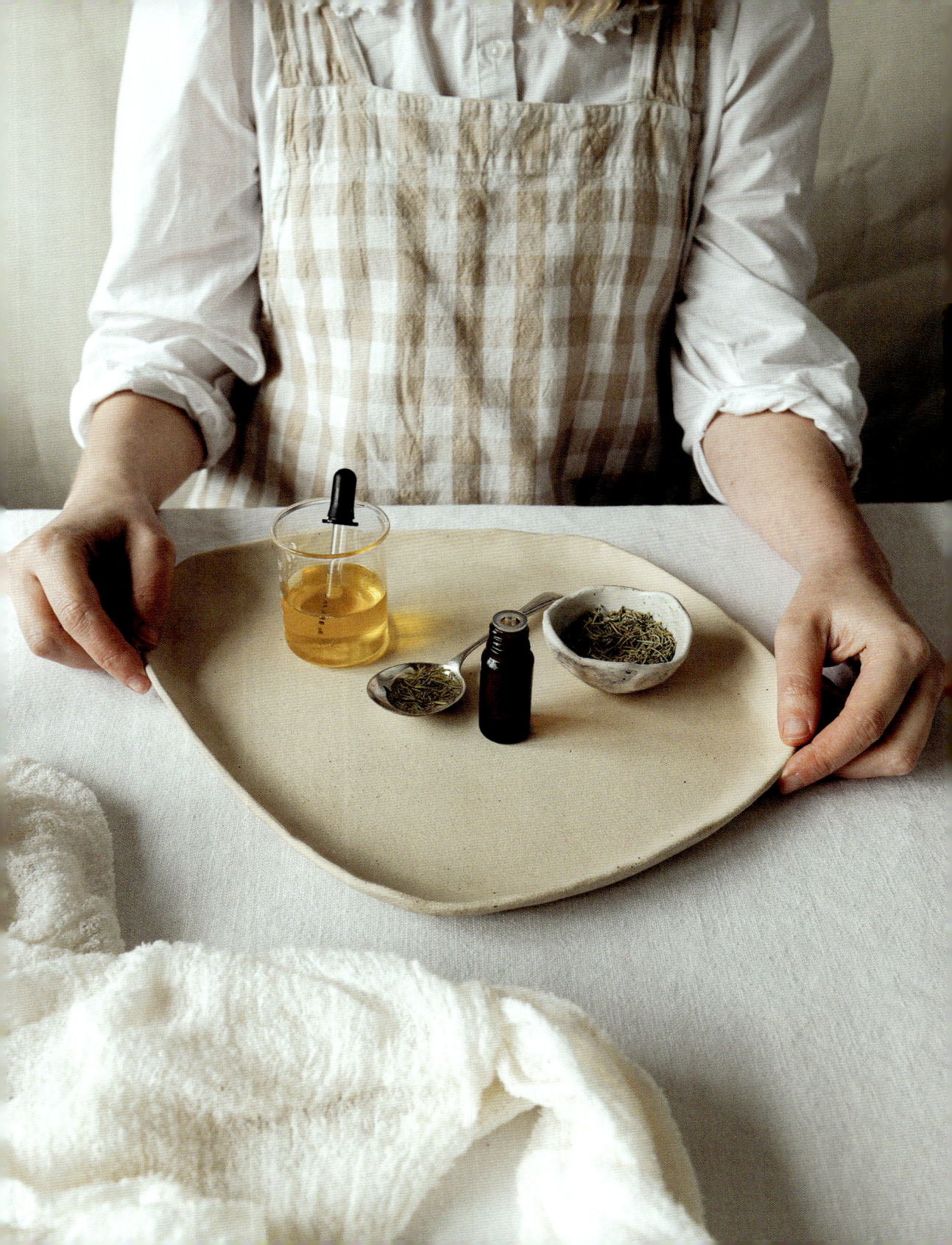

# EYEBROW GROWTH OIL

*I have to admit that being a millennial I fell victim to overplucking my eyebrows when I was younger, and I deeply regret this stage of my life. I created this eyebrow oil to help repair some of the damage that occurred over the years, and it helps to make my brows feel thicker and stronger. The added benefit is that it's packed full of rosemary, which is one of my favorite fragrances.*

*Makes* 1 small bottle (20 ml [⅛ cup])

14 g (3 tsp) castor oil
5 g (1 tsp) Rosemary Infused Oil (page 123)
0.2 g rosemary essential oil

In a bowl, combine the castor oil, Rosemary Infused Oil and rosemary essential oil.

Transfer to a small sterile bottle. Dispense just a drop at a time. Massage the eyebrows with just one drop of oil as part of your evening skin care routine.

## Get to Know Your Ingredients!

Rosemary is a superpower in hair care. It strengthens hair, making it more resistant to damage, and is also known to strengthen roots, improve circulation and prevent hair loss.

# NOURISHING CUTICLE BALM

*I decided to make a cuticle balm instead of an oil because I like to make it part of my nighttime rituals, to be kept on the bedside table and massaged into my cuticles before I fall asleep. This balm will also help to strengthen your nails for pampered and protected hands.*

*Makes* 2 small tins (24 g [0.5 oz] each)

10 g (3 tsp) cocoa butter
6 g (1 tsp) Calendula Infused Oil (page 120)
6 g (1 tsp) castor oil
2 g beeswax
0.2 g vitamin E oil
0.2 g mandarin essential oil
0.1 g clove essential oil

Using the double boiler method, gently melt the cocoa butter, Calendula Infused Oil, castor oil and beeswax until it is a liquid consistency. Read more about the double boiler method on page 146.

Take the mixture off the heat and place it in the refrigerator. When the mixture has cooled to below 105°F (40°C), add the vitamin E oil, mandarin essential oil and clove essential oil. This should only take 5 minutes to cool. Stir to combine.

Transfer to your containers and label. Massage a pea-sized amount into your cuticles at night as a daily treatment.

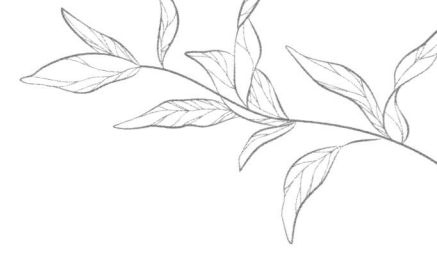

## Get to Know Your Ingredients!

The cocoa butter and beeswax help to soften the cuticles and form a protective layer over the skin, keeping moisture locked in for longer and allowing for the ingredients to penetrate and treat the skin.

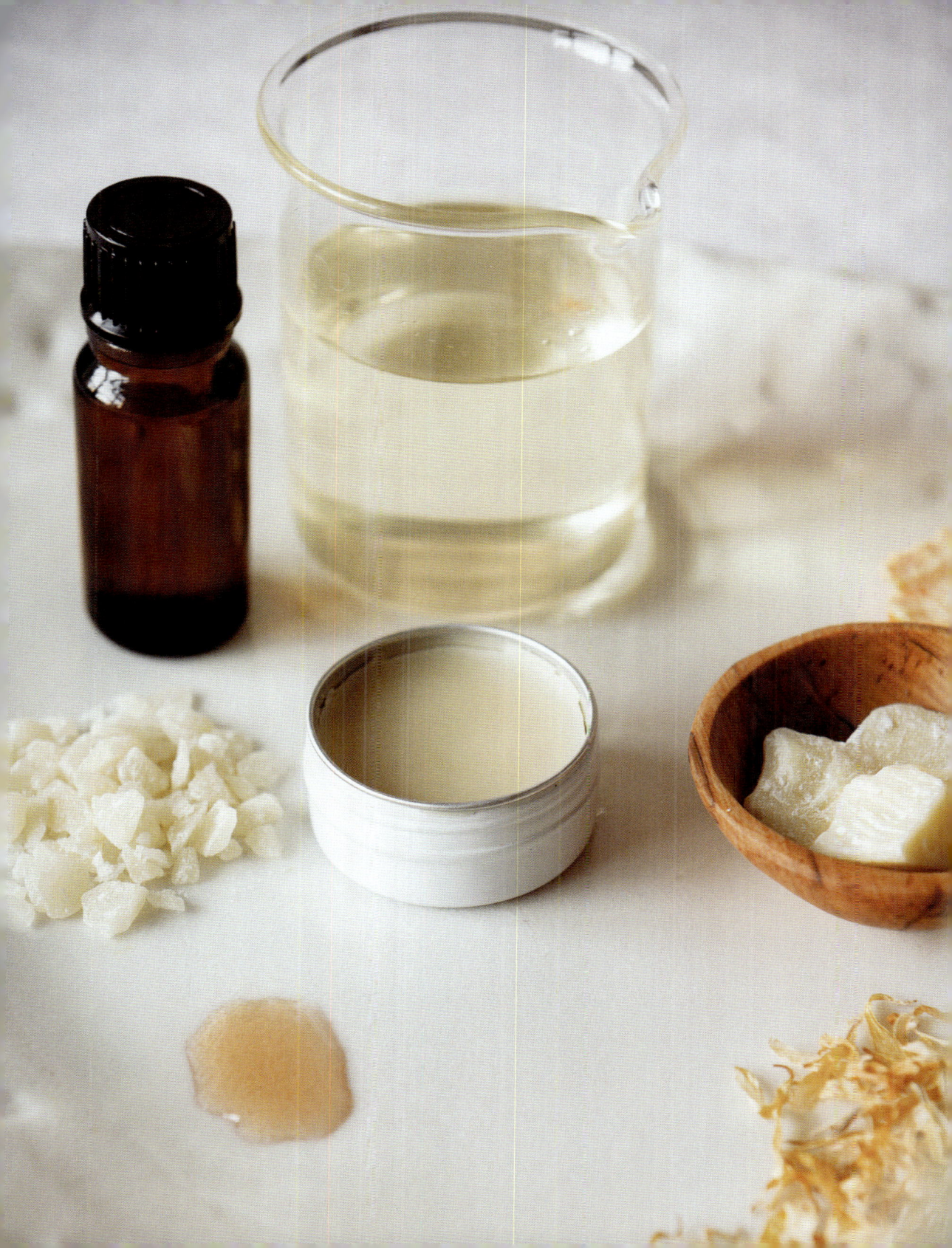

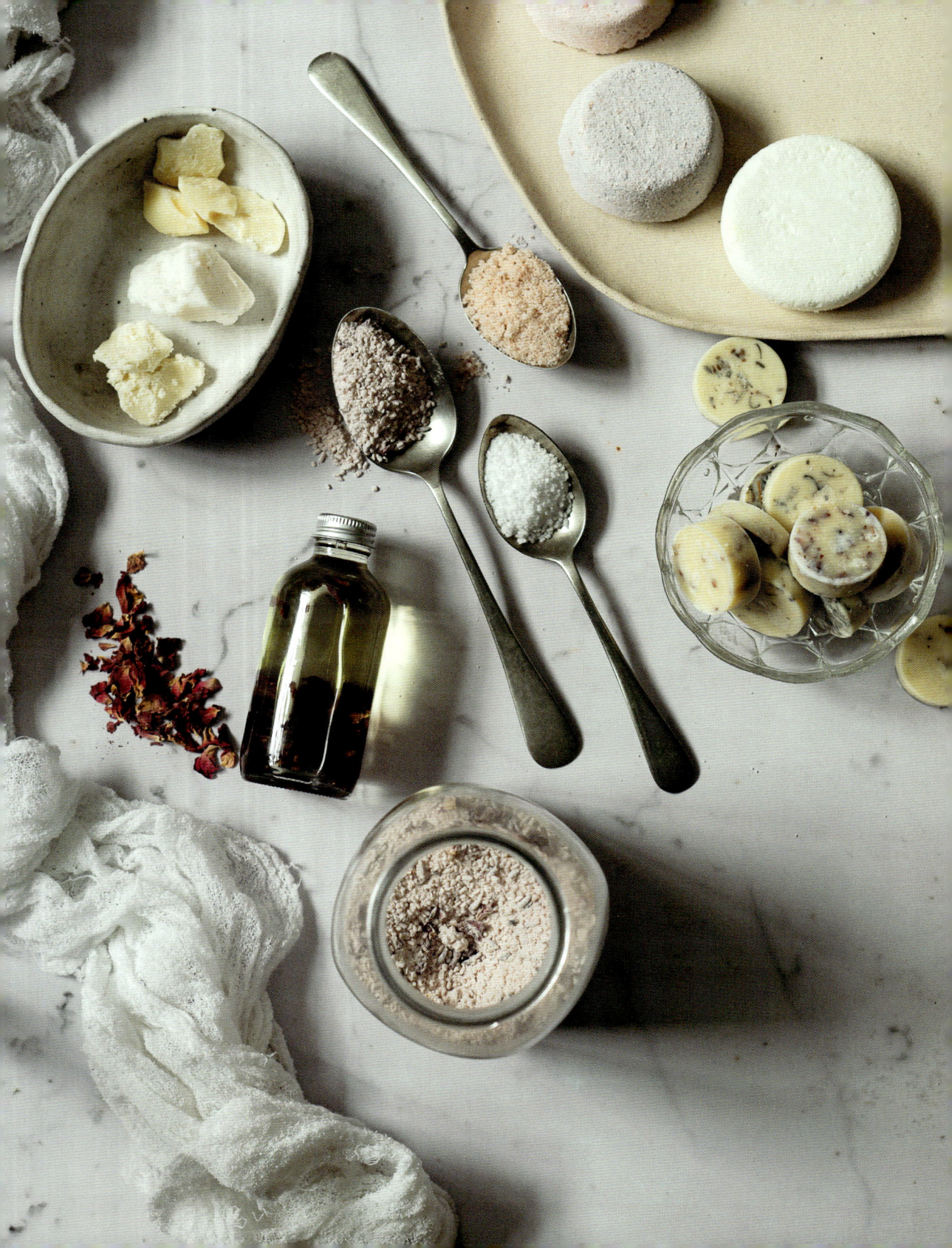

# BATH INDULGENCE

It's time for a little bit of rest and relaxation, and I have the most wonderful recipes to share with you that will help to melt away the day's stress and enjoy a little bit of me time. All of these recipes would also make beautiful gifts for someone special!

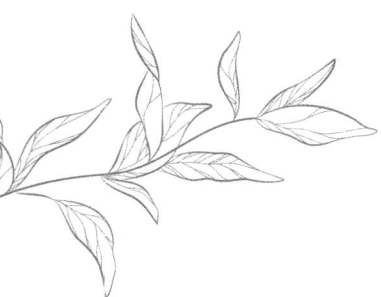

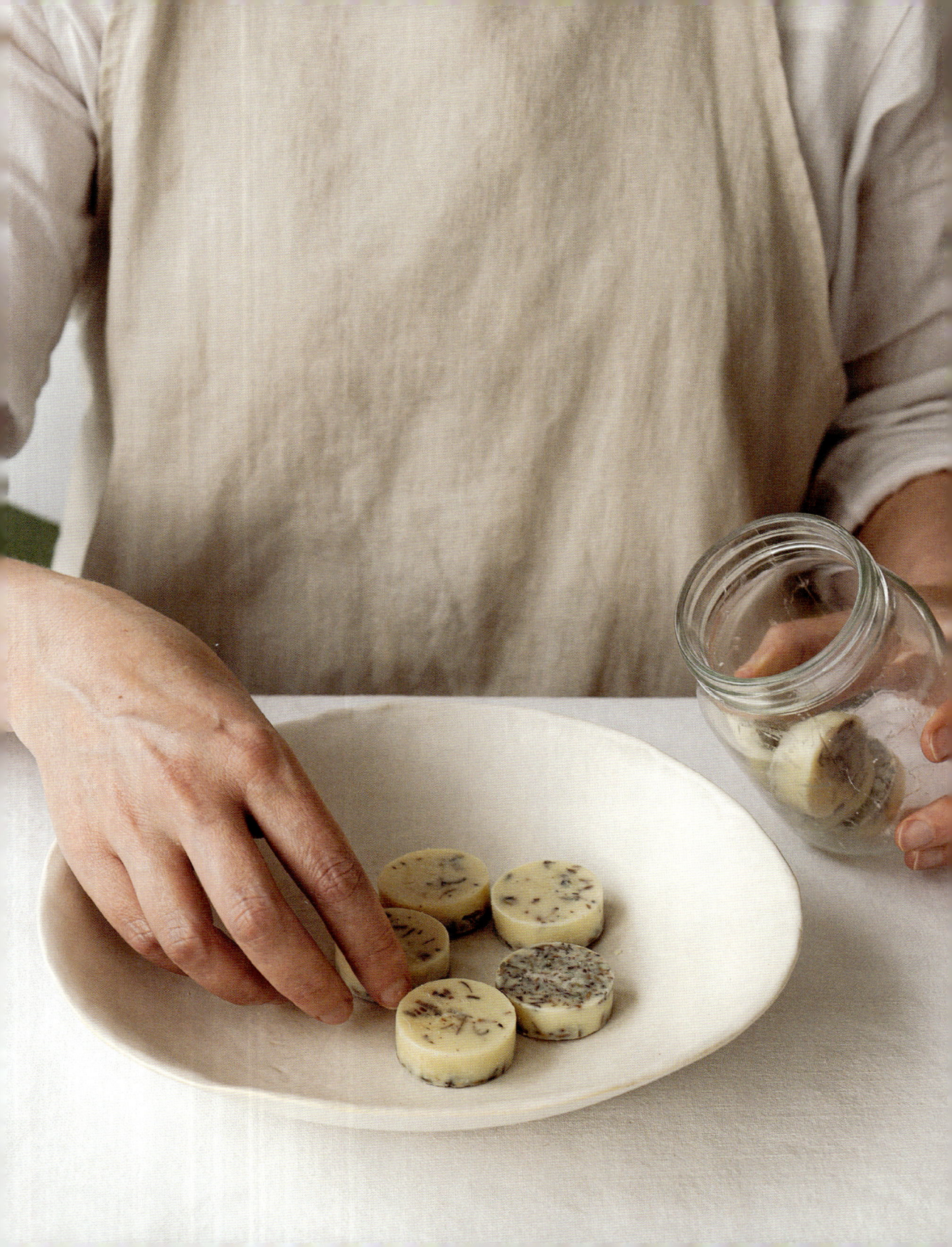

# CALMING BATH MELTS

*If you haven't tried a bath melt yet, you are in for a treat! When added to your water, these soothing bath melts will release the beautiful butters and oils, nourishing your skin as you bathe. The essential oils also create a wonderful relaxing atmosphere, which helps to turn your bath into a soothing spa-like moment.*

*Makes* about 9 bath melts

65 g (4 tbsp) cocoa butter

18 g (1½ tbsp) apricot kernel oil

10 g (3 tsp) Calendula Infused Oil (page 120)

2 g lavender buds

1.1 g lavender essential oil

1 g vitamin E oil

0.5 g geranium essential oil

0.4 g bergamot essential oil

Using the double boiler method, gently melt the cocoa butter, apricot kernel oil and Calendula Infused Oil until it is a liquid consistency. Read more about the double boiler method on page 146.

Take the mixture off the heat and place in the refrigerator. When the mixture has cooled to below 105°F (40°C), add the lavender buds, lavender essential oil, vitamin E oil, geranium essential oil and bergamot essential oil. This should take 10 to 15 minutes to cool. Stir to combine.

Pour into silicone molds of your choice. I like to use small molds that are approximately 4 centimeters (1½ inches) wide and 1 centimeter (½ inch) deep. Place in the fridge to set.

Store in an airtight container. Drop into a warm bathwater for a deeply relaxing bath experience.

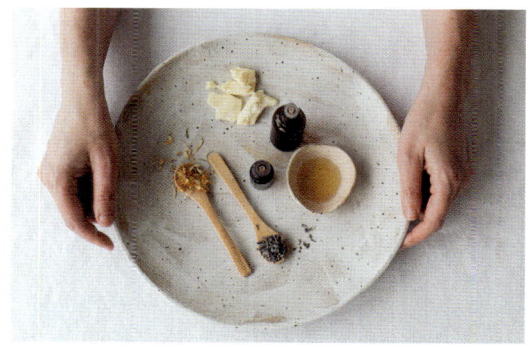

## Get to Know Your Ingredients!

Cocoa butter is deeply moisturizing and contains antioxidants, including vitamin E. Regular use helps to maintain your skin's elasticity and can also help even your skin tone.

The combination of lavender and bergamot essential oils in this recipe is both relaxing and rejuvenating to provide you with that perfect moment of relaxation while you bathe.

# UPLIFTING BATH MELTS

*This bath melt recipe combines both uplifting and anxiety-reducing fragrances to fully prepare you for the day. Just run it under warm water and step into the bath for an uplifting moment.*

*Makes* 9 bath melts

65 g (4 tbsp) cocoa butter
17 g (1½ tbsp) sweet almond oil
10 g (3 tsp) Rosehip Infused Oil (page 128)
2 g rose petals
1 g vitamin E oil
1 g mandarin essential oil
1 g rosemary essential oil

Using the double boiler method, gently melt the cocoa butter, sweet almond oil and Rosehip Infused Oil until it is a liquid consistency. Read more about the double boiler method on page 146.

Take off the heat and place in the refrigerator. When the mixture has cooled to below 105°F (40°C), add the rose petals, vitamin E oil, mandarin essential oil and rosemary essential oil. This should take 10 to 15 minutes to cool. Stir to combine.

Pour into silicone molds of your choice. I like to use small molds that are approximately 4 centimeters (1½ inches) wide and 1 centimeter (½ inch) deep. Place in the fridge to set.

Store in an airtight container. Drop into warm bathwater for a deeply soothing bath.

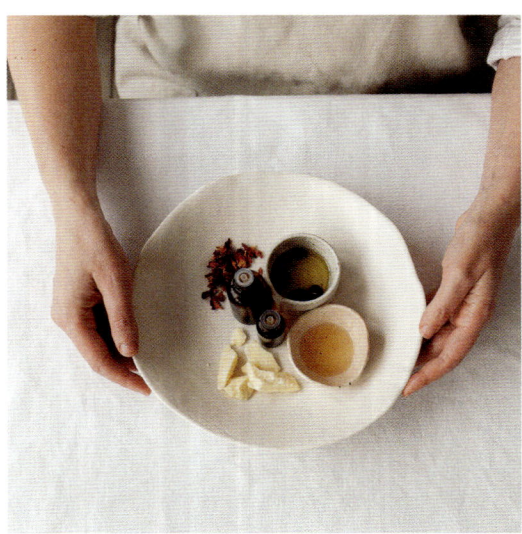

## Get to Know Your Ingredients!

The butters and oils in this recipe are rich in vitamins A, D, K and E, which all contribute to overall skin health. Your skin care products are even working for you when you're taking a bath!

I have added botanicals to both of these recipes. They are a beautiful addition to these recipes, but if you'd like to leave them out because you prefer your bath without the addition of them, then you absolutely can!

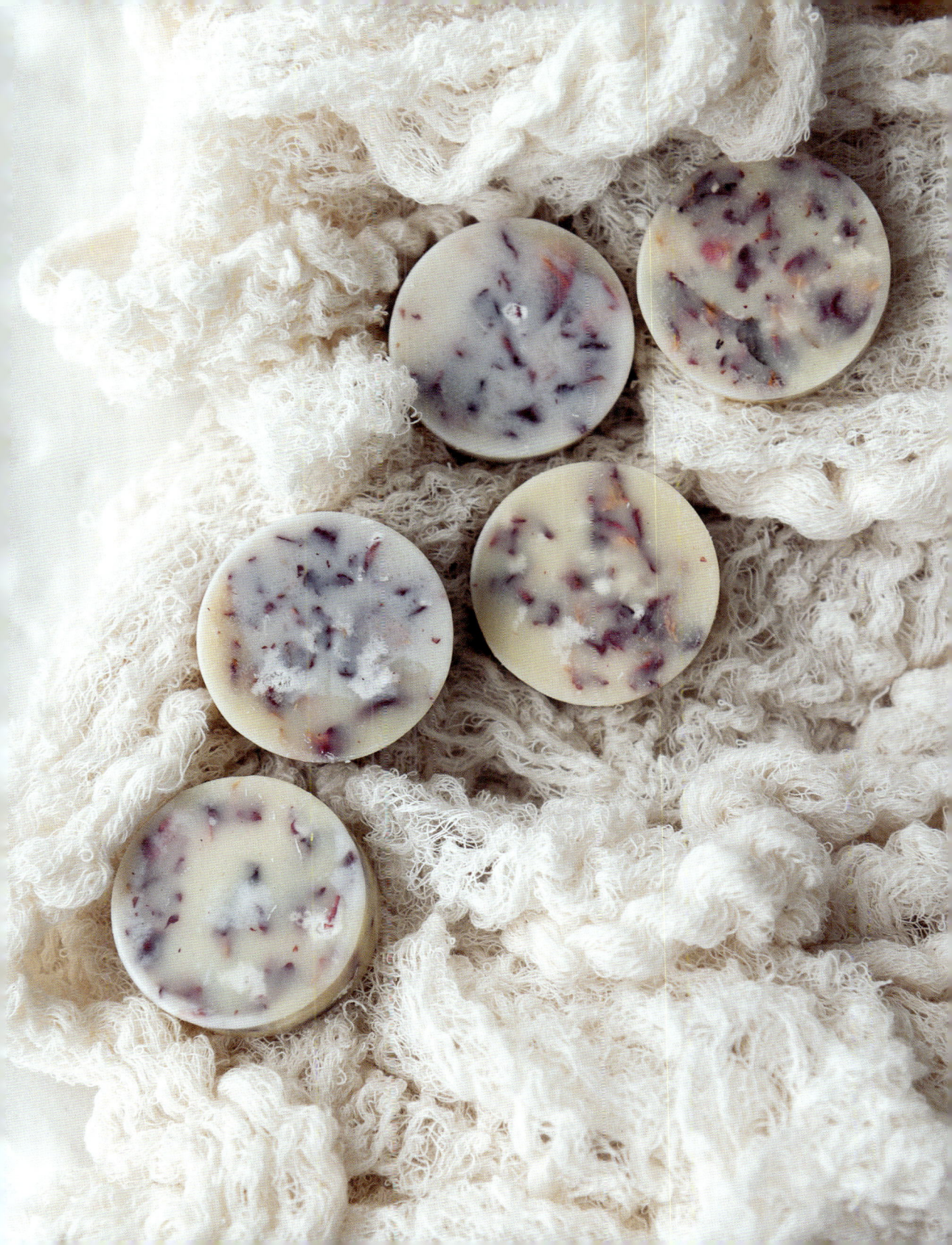

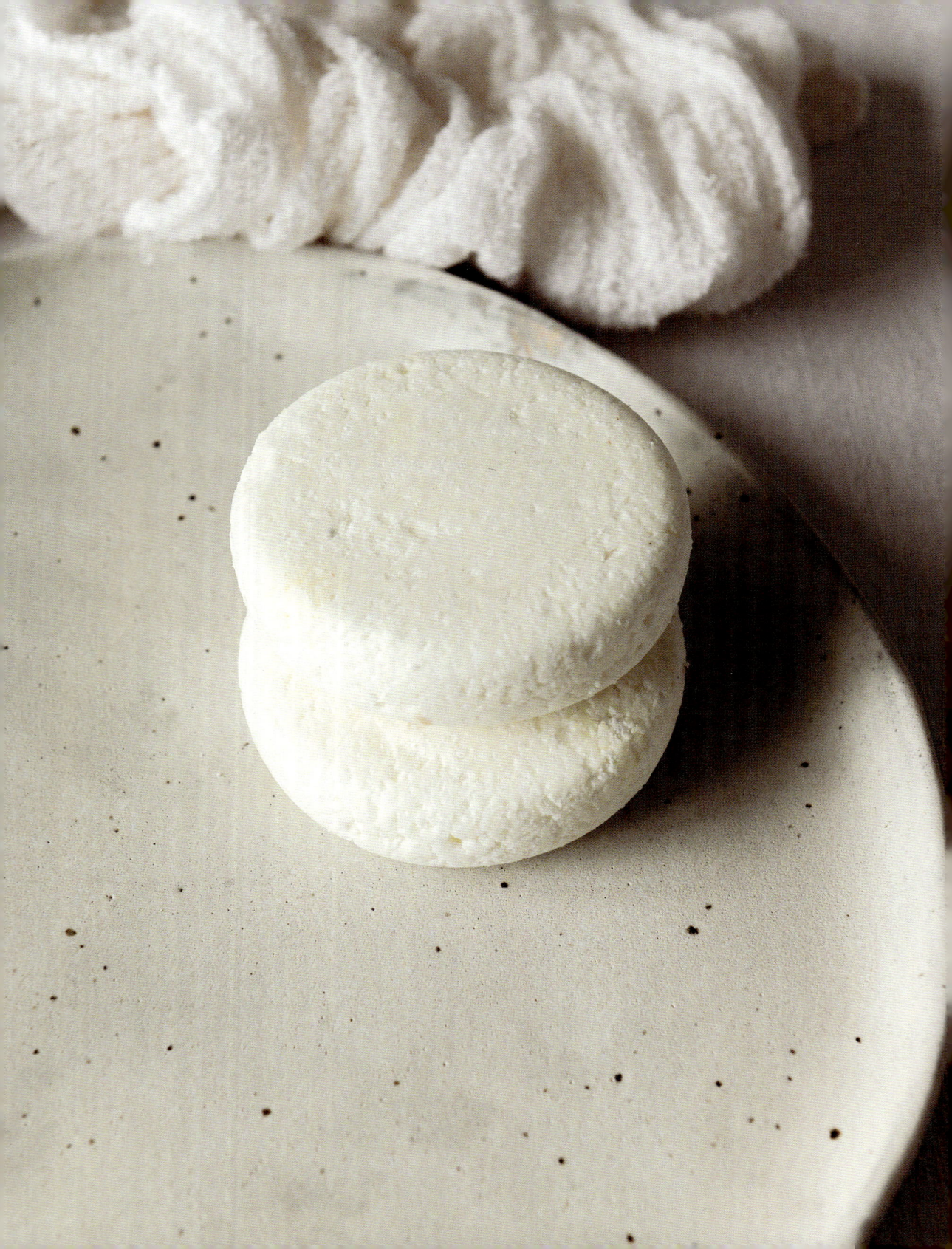

# RELAX AND UNWIND BATH BOMBS

*Who doesn't love the joy of a bath bomb? What might surprise you is that as well as the theater that a bath bomb provides, it is also very good for your skin!*

*Makes* 2 large bath bombs

100 g (1 cup) baking soda

50 g (½ cup) citric acid

25 g (¼ cup) cornflour (cornstarch)

25 g (2 tbsp) Epsom salt

25 g (2 tbsp) coconut oil

0.5 g lavender essential oil

0.5 g geranium essential oil

0.2 g clove essential oil

Water, from a spray bottle

Place the baking soda, citric acid, cornflour and Epsom salt in a bowl and stir to combine.

Melt the coconut oil using the double boiler method until liquid. Read more about the double boiler method on page 146.

Slowly add the coconut oil to the dry mixture and stir to combine. Add the lavender essential oil, geranium essential oil and clove essential oil.

When fully combined, spray a small amount of water over the mixture and continue mixing. You will only need to spray this once or twice to get the consistency you need. Your mixture should appear like wet sand and start clumping together when it is ready for the molds.

Add to molds of your choice. You can use silicone or aluminum molds in any shape you choose. Drop into your bathwater on those days that you just need a little TLC.

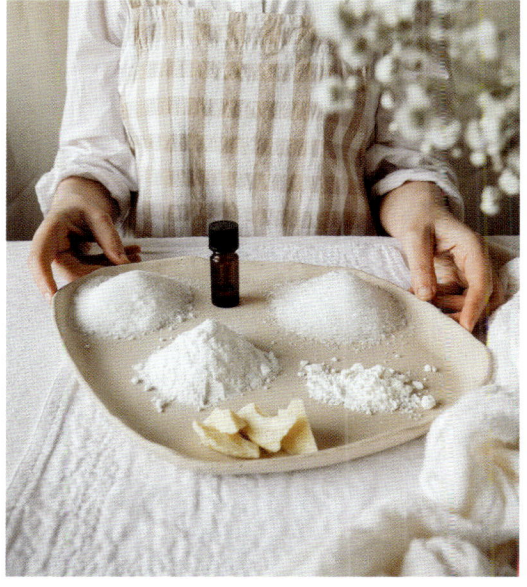

## Get to Know Your Ingredients!

Bath bombs offer such a relaxing bathing experience and just add that little extra luxury to your bathing routine. I have added coconut oil to this recipe, as it nourishes the skin while you bathe and leaves your skin feeling soft and moisturized.

The baking soda and cornflour in this recipe help to soften your bathwater and soften and soothe your skin. I live in the U.K., where cornflour is a silky white powder, not yellow, so don't be confused! In the United States and Canada, the word that one uses for this ingredient is cornstarch.

# LOVELY BUBBLES BATH BOMBS

*I whip up a batch of these bath bombs with the help of my children, who love experimenting and making lots of different colors! I make smaller bombs for their little hands and also reuse a muffin tin to make the molds for them. Have fun with them, as they can be as rustic as you like. They also work well with botanicals if you want to add them in too! Of course, they are also completely suitable for children to use in the bath.*

*Makes* 6 medium-sized bath bombs

200 g (2 cups) baking soda
100 g (1 cup) citric acid
50 g (½ cup) cornflour (cornstarch)
50 g (4 tbsp) Epsom salt
1 g natural food coloring of your choice
50 g (3 tbsp) coconut oil
Water, from a spray bottle

Place the baking soda, citric acid, cornflour and Epsom salt in a bowl and stir to combine.

Add the natural food coloring of your choice and stir in. You can get as creative as you like here! Stirring in just a little can create a lovely marble effect or adding more than one color can make them look tie-dyed!

Melt the coconut oil using the double boiler method until liquid. Read more about the double boiler method on page 146.

Slowly add the coconut oil to the dry mixture and stir to combine.

When fully combined, spray a small amount of water over the mixture and continue mixing. You will only need to spray this once or twice to get the consistency you need. Your mixture should appear like wet sand and start clumping together when it is ready for the molds.

Add to molds of your choice. I use a muffin baking tray for these bath bombs, but you can use silicone or aluminum molds in any shape you choose. Add to your bathwater and enjoy the lovely bubbles!

## Get to Know Your Ingredients!

I don't use essential oils when making bath bombs for my children. Some essential oils aren't suitable for children under a certain age, with essential oils like peppermint and eucalyptus being too strong for children.

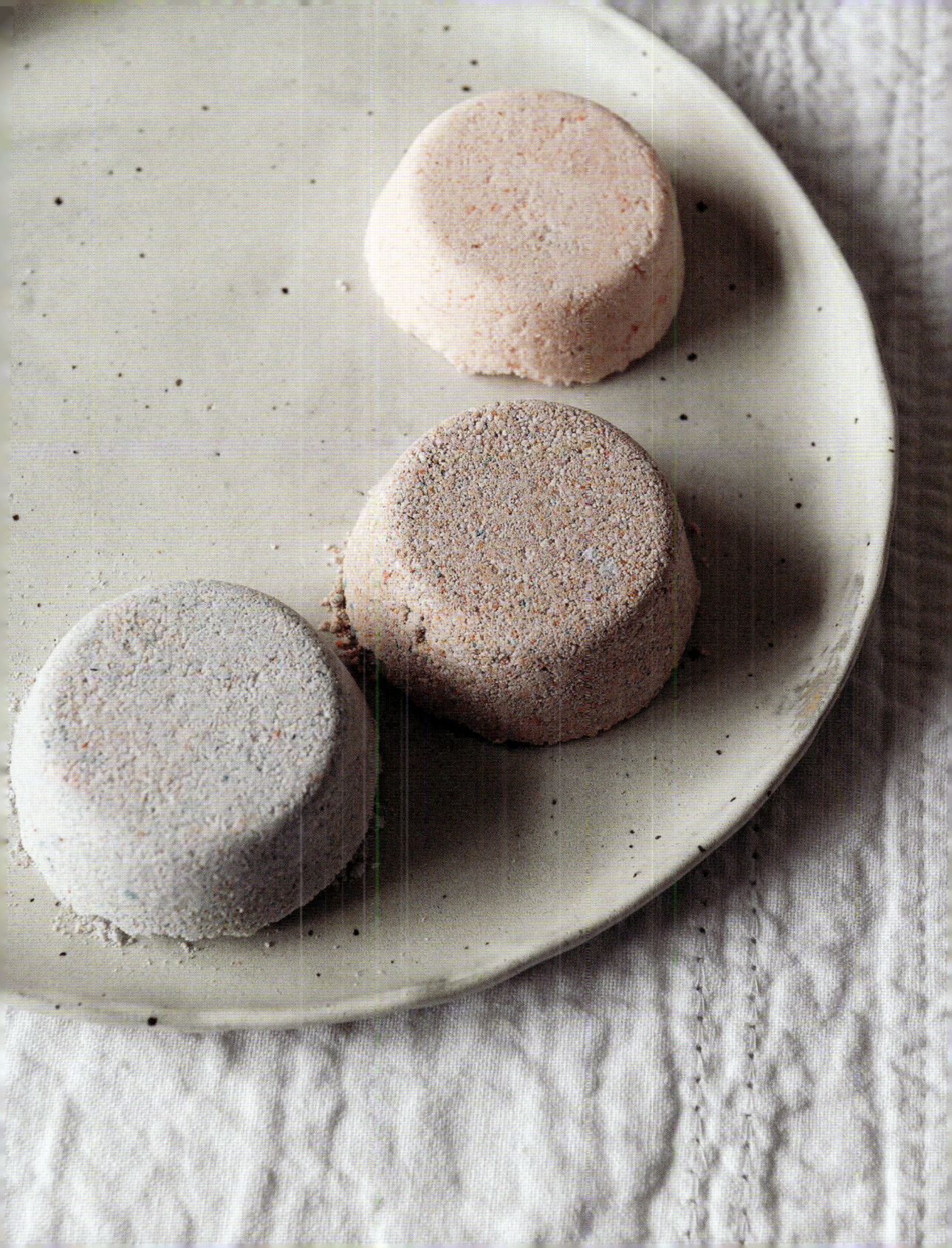

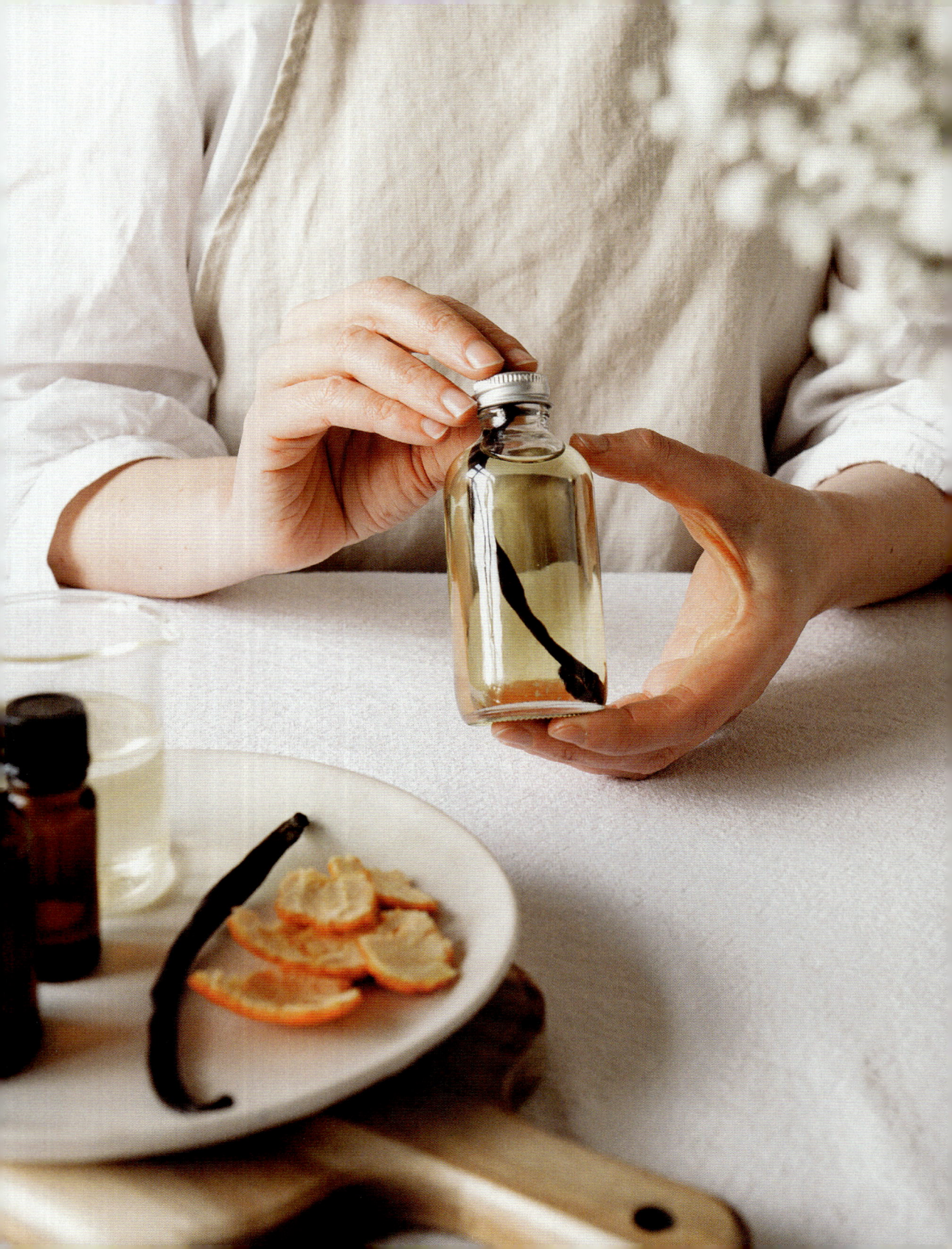

# SOOTHING BATH AND BODY OIL

*I absolutely love using these oils on my skin. They are an all-natural way to moisturize your skin, one of the simplest recipes to make and are multipurpose too. I like to use about a teaspoon to rub into my skin after a shower to keep it nourished and hydrated or add a teaspoon to my bathwater to nourish my skin while I bathe.*

*Makes* 1 medium bottle (200 ml [¾ cup])

100 g (5½ tbsp) grapeseed oil
50 g (3 tbsp) sweet almond oil
47 g (3 tbsp) apricot kernel oil
1.5 g vitamin E oil
1 g mandarin essential oil
0.5 g peppermint essential oil
1 vanilla pod

Add the grapeseed oil, sweet almond oil, apricot kernel oil, vitamin E oil, mandarin essential oil and peppermint essential oil to a bowl and stir to thoroughly combine.

Transfer to a clean, sterile bottle. Add the vanilla pod to your bottle.

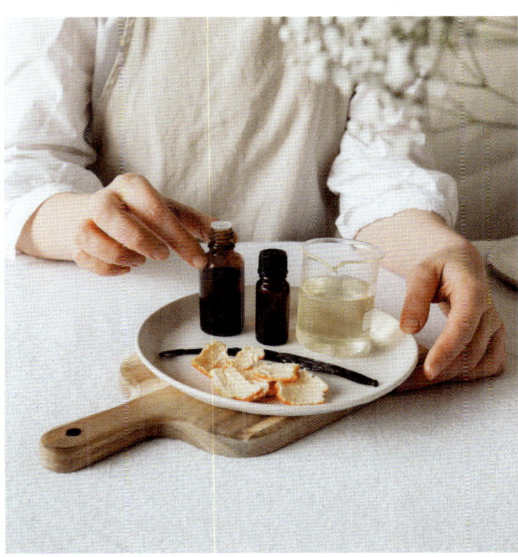

### Get to Know Your Ingredients!

I have added a vanilla pod to this recipe. It's one of my favorite fragrances but also has benefits in skin care and contains antioxidant properties. I like to refill this bottle and keep the vanilla pod and reuse it every time I fill the bottle up. The vanilla pod should last for six months when used in this way.

Grapeseed oil is a great moisturizer for the skin and doesn't leave it feeling greasy. It is also rich in antioxidants.

# BOTANICAL BATH AND BODY OIL

*This is another beautiful bath and body oil that I love to use. I have included my favorite infusions and fragrances in this recipe to make a beautiful and aromatic oil. It's one of my favorite ways to relax and unwind while bathing and also prepares my skin for the day when used after a shower.*

*Makes* 1 medium bottle (200 ml [¾ cup])

100 g (6½ tbsp) sweet almond oil

80 g (4½ tbsp) apricot kernel oil

9 g (3 tsp) Rosehip Infused Oil (page 128)

9 g (3 tsp) Lavender Infused Oil (page 119)

1 g lavender essential oil

0.5 g geranium essential oil

0.5 g rose petals

Add the sweet almond oil, apricot kernel oil, Rosehip Infused Oil, Lavender Infused Oil, lavender essential oil, geranium essential oil and rose petals to a bowl and stir to thoroughly combine.

Transfer the mixture to a clean, sterile bottle.

Add a teaspoon to your running bathwater or rub a teaspoon over your skin after a shower for nourished skin.

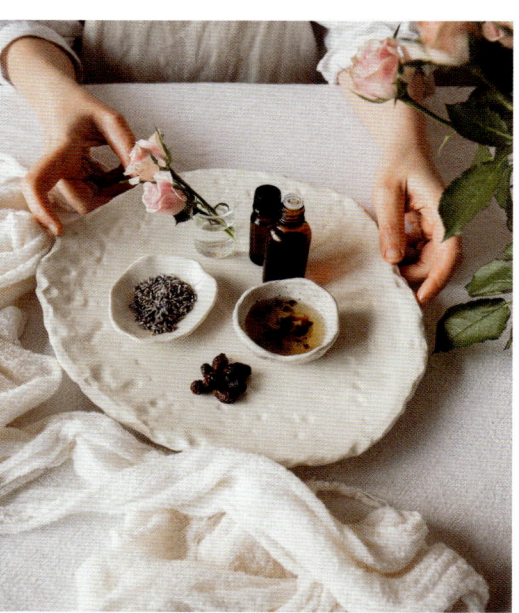

## Get to Know Your Ingredients!

The apricot kernel oil in this recipe is rich in oleic and linoleic acids, which help to maintain the skin's barrier function. It's a popular oil to help soothe sensitive and dry skin and provides moisturization without feeling heavy.

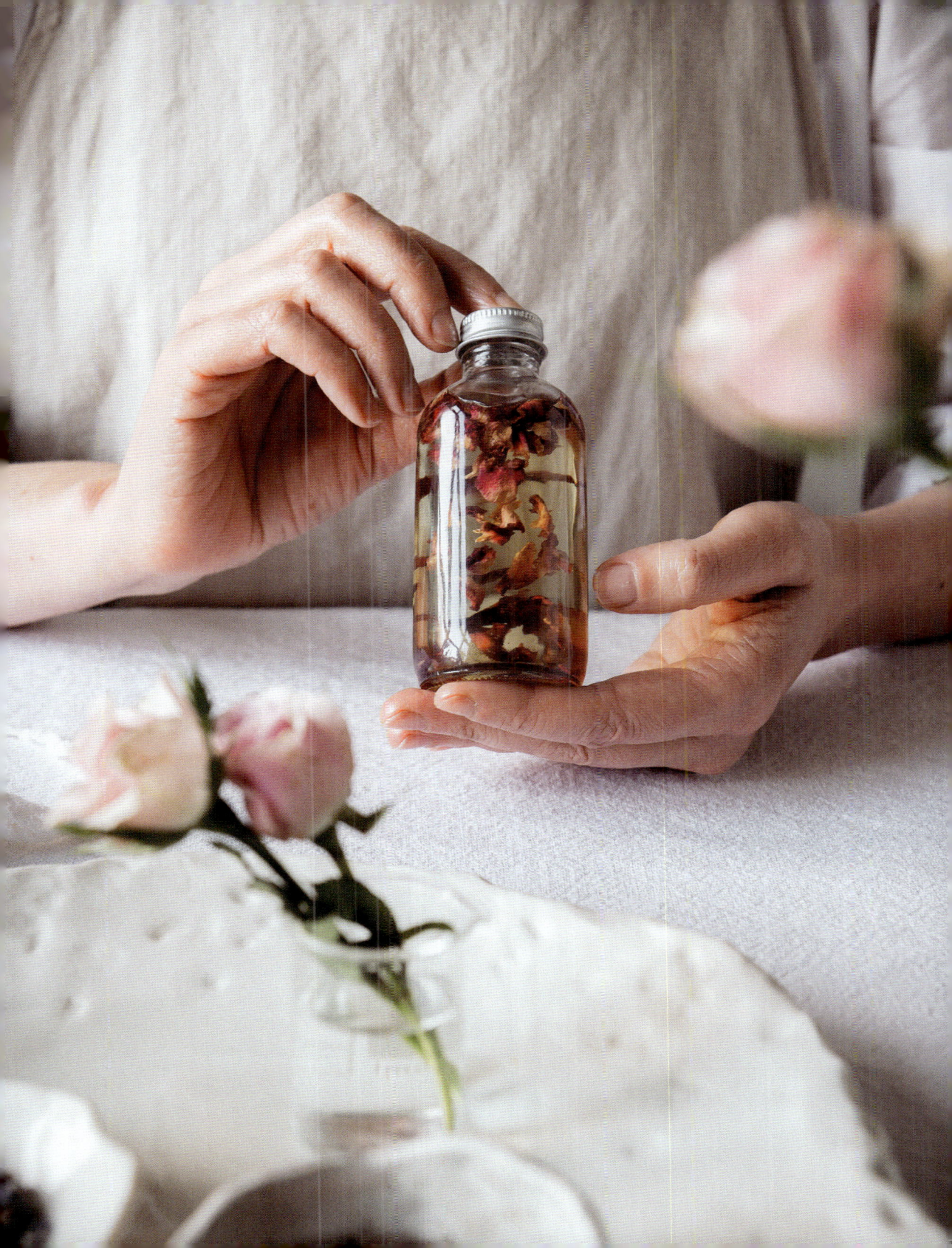

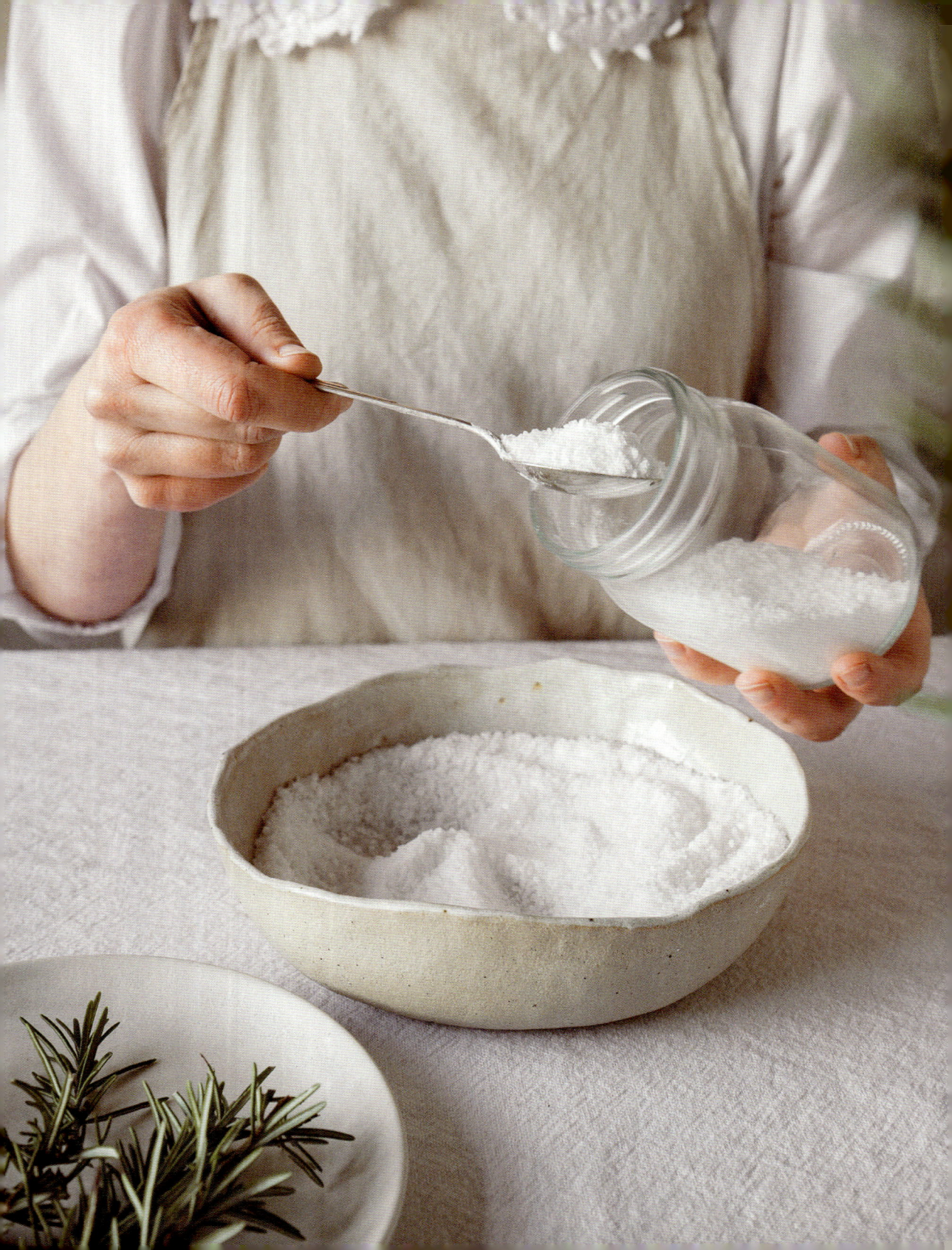

# HERBAL INFUSED BATH SALTS

*These herbal bath salts are rich in minerals, deeply relaxing and will help to relieve the day's tension. Add to your bathwater for a deeply relaxing and restorative bath.*

*Makes* 1 extra-large jar (750 g [6 cups])

600 g (3 cups) Epsom salt
100 g (1 cup) baking soda
3 g (1 tsp) rosemary essential oil
1.5 g clary sage essential oil
1.5 g bergamot essential oil
1 g clove essential oil

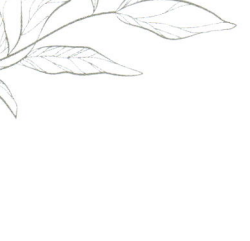

In a large bowl, thoroughly combine the Epsom salt and baking soda. Add the rosemary essential oil, clary sage essential oil, bergamot essential oil and clove essential oil.

Transfer to a large, clean jar.

Scoop up to 1 cup (about 125 g) into your bathwater. Relax and enjoy!

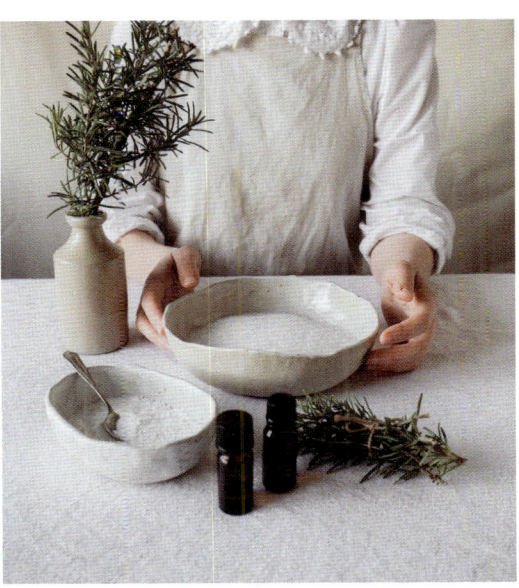

## Get to Know Your Ingredients!

Epsom salt is a beautiful way to relax and unwind after a long day. They are rich in magnesium and help to alleviate muscle soreness.

Soaking in an Epsom salt bath before bedtime can also contribute to better sleep, promote stress relief and relaxation and help the body to detoxify.

Bath Indulgence

# FLORAL BATH SALTS

*These floral bath salts are a beautiful way to relax and unwind. The fragrance is uplifting and the ingredients help to soften your skin and soothe your body.*

*Makes* 1 extra-large jar (750 g [6 cups])

600 g (3 cups) Epsom salt
90 g (1 cup) baking soda
40 g (2 cups) pink kaolin clay
8 g (1 tbsp) lavender flowers
8 g (1 tbsp) rose petals
1 g lavender essential oil
1 g geranium essential oil
1 g bergamot essential oil
1 g chamomile essential oil

In a large bowl, thoroughly combine the Epsom salt, baking soda, pink kaolin clay, lavender flowers and rose petals. Add the lavender essential oil, geranium essential oil, bergamot essential oil and chamomile essential oil.

Transfer to a clean, large jar.

Scoop up to 1 cup (about 125 g) into your bathwater. Relax and enjoy!

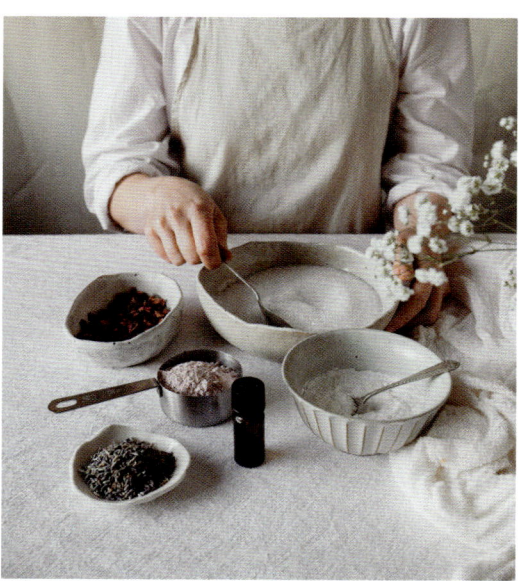

## Get to Know Your Ingredients!

As well as the deeply soothing Epsom salt, kaolin clay has natural detoxifying properties, which help draw out impurities while also helping to soothe your skin.

I love to add botanicals to my bath salts to display them and add to my bathwater. However, if you are worried about them going down your drain, I have a great solution! I add a scoop to a small cotton bag and add this to my bathwater. The contents infuse in the bath while keeping the botanicals away from the drain.

The Natural Skin Care Recipe Book

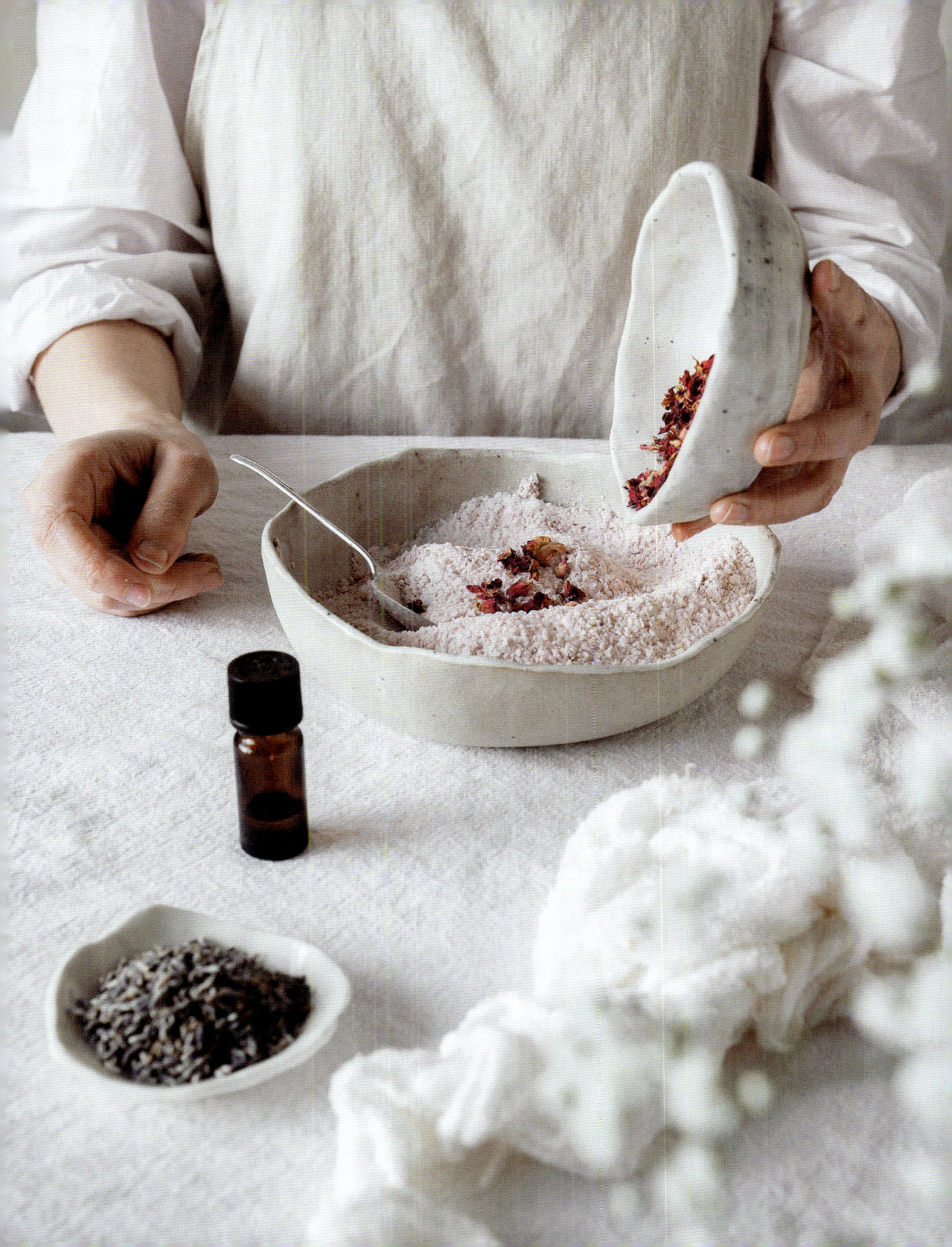

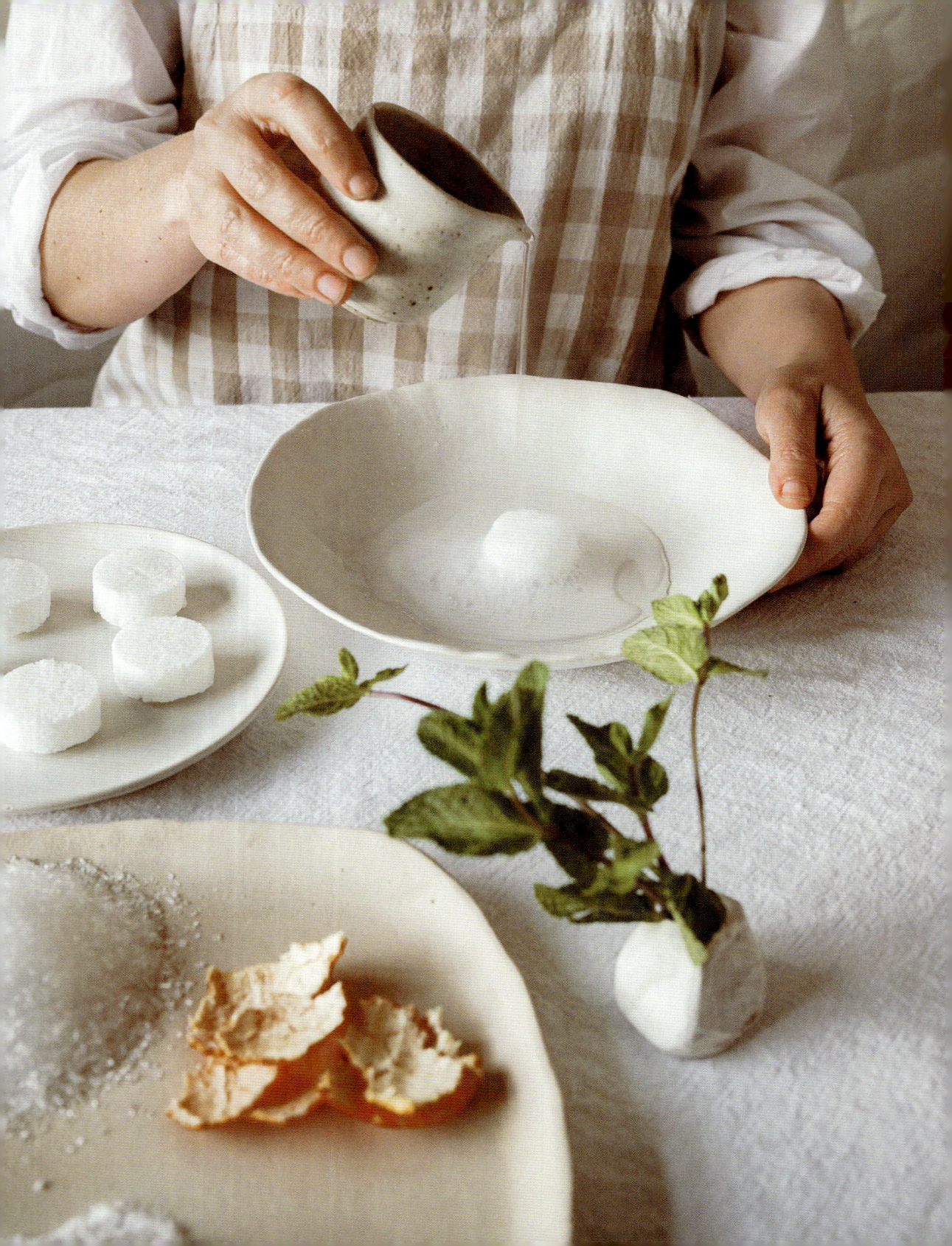

# WAKE UP SHOWER STEAMERS

*I make these shower steamers similarly to the bath bombs. They're really simple to use, and instead of placing them in the bathtub, you place them on the floor of your shower. When they are placed in the shower, the aromatherapy of the essential oils is dispersed into the air. These shower steamers have been made with essential oils that help wake you up and uplift you in the morning.*

*Makes* 9 shower steamers

32 g (⅓ cup) baking soda
32 g (⅓ cup) citric acid
32 g (2½ tbsp) Epsom salt
2 g peppermint essential oil
2 g mandarin essential oil
2 g tea tree essential oil
Water, from a spray bottle

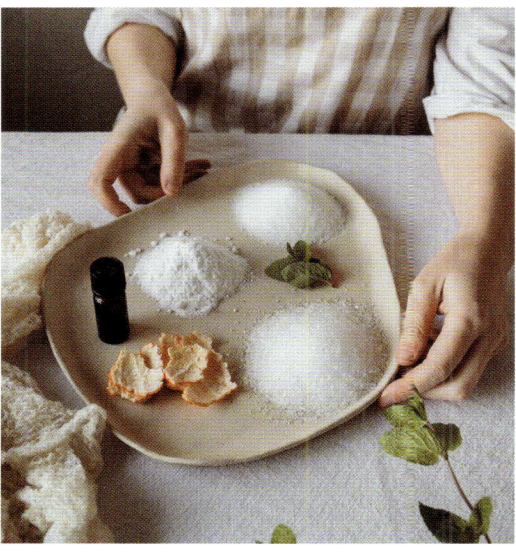

Place the baking soda, citric acid and Epsom salt in a bowl and stir to combine.

Add the peppermint essential oil, mandarin essential oil and tea tree essential oil to a bowl and stir to combine. Slowly add this to the dry mixture.

When fully combined, spray a small amount of water to the mixture (you will only need one to two sprays) and continue mixing together. Your mixture should appear like wet sand and start clumping together when it is ready for the molds.

Add the mixture to small molds. I like to use molds that are 4 centimeters (1½ inches) wide and 1 centimeter (½ inch) deep in size, so that I can add one to my shower in the morning to help me wake up!

## Get to Know Your Ingredients!

I chose to use mandarin, peppermint and tea tree essential oils when making these shower steamers. The mandarin is uplifting and mood enhancing. The peppermint is energizing and helps to improve concentration. The tea tree is a natural decongestant. Combined, these ingredients are sure to begin your day the right way.

You will need to add just a spray or two to this recipe to set the shower steamers in the molds. Don't overestimate how much you need; as soon as the mixture feels like wet sand, stop adding the water. If it starts excessively foaming, it makes the mixture very unstable and difficult to set.

# SLEEPY TIME SHOWER STEAMERS

*These shower steamers are sure to help you relax and unwind after a long day. They combine my favorite stress-relieving fragrances.*

*Makes* 9 shower steamers

32 g (⅓ cup) baking soda
32 g (⅓ cup) citric acid
32 g (2½ tbsp) Epsom salt
2 g lavender essential oil
2 g rosemary essential oil
2 g clary sage essential oil
Water, from a spray bottle

Place the baking soda, citric acid and Epsom salt in a bowl and stir to combine.

Add the lavender essential oil, rosemary essential oil and clary sage essential oil to a bowl and stir to combine. Slowly add this to the dry mixture.

When fully combined, spray a small amount of water to the mixture and continue mixing. You will only need one to two sprays. Your mixture should appear like wet sand and start clumping together when it is ready for the molds.

Add to small molds. I like to use molds that are 4 centimeters (1½ inches) wide and 1 centimeter (½ inch) deep in size, so that I can add one to my shower after a long day to help me relax and unwind.

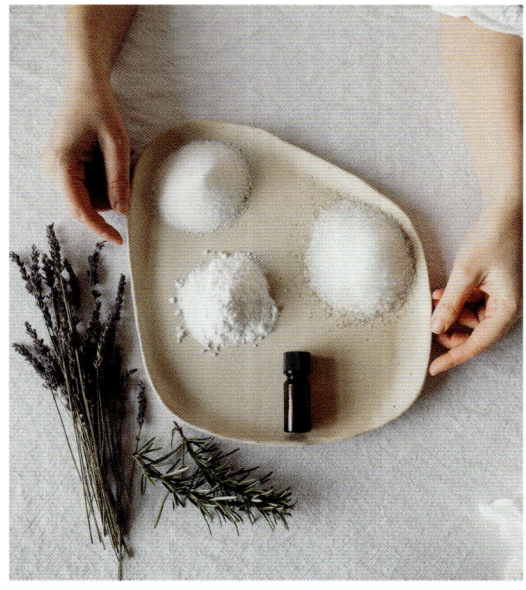

## Get to Know Your Ingredients!

I chose lavender, rosemary and clary sage essential oils for these shower steamers. The lavender is relaxing and a natural stress reliever; the rosemary is also a natural stress reliever and is used to relieve headaches; and clary sage is known to help regulate hormonal balance.

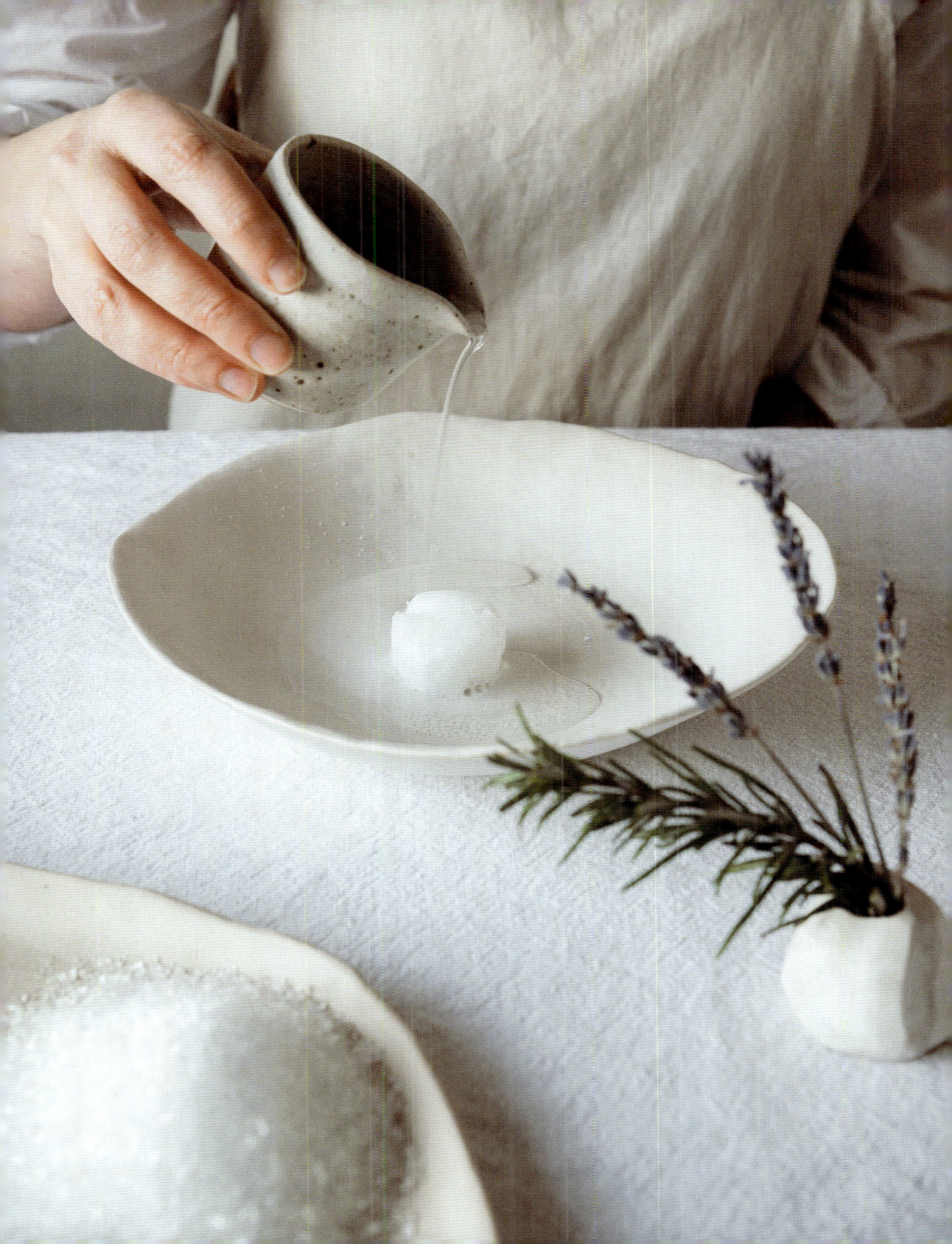

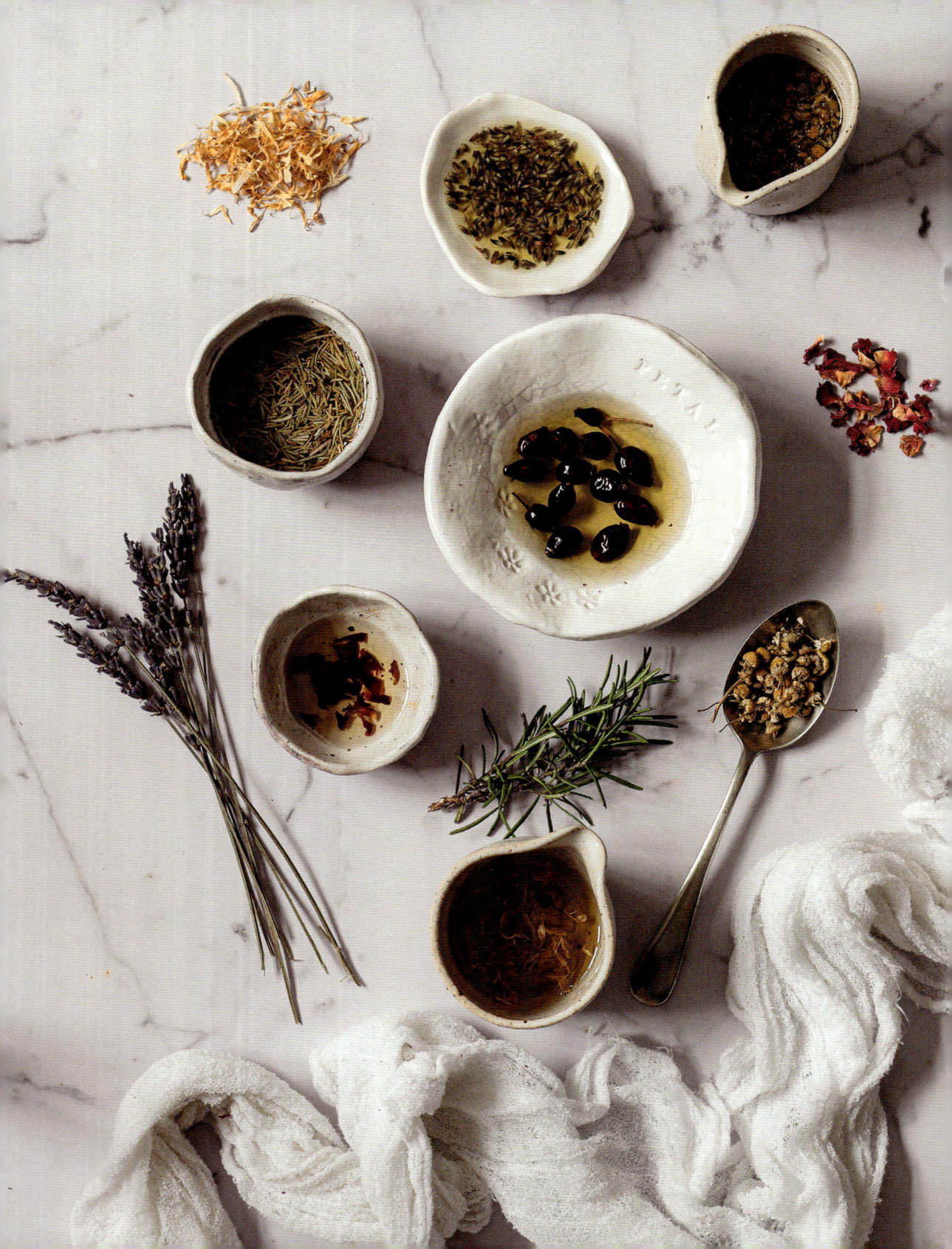

# BOTANICAL OILS

You will see that the majority of the recipes I have included in this skin care guide contain botanical oils. These are my favorite ingredients to use. I find the process of infusing botanical oils is not only fun but really helps you to connect to the product that you are making and the ingredients you are using. It's not a sweeping statement to say that all of the botanicals I use within this skin care guide are deeply restorative, but you will find that their properties are so healing and soothing.

This is the part of the skin care guide where you can really start experimenting. When you make all of the different skin care recipes, feel free to experiment and swap one infused oil for another depending on your preferences. If you find that you have a favorite botanical, you can add it to every recipe that you make!

I have also created these recipes without specifying which carrier oil you add to your essential oils to because the choice is yours. I will include five options below that will behave very similarly in the recipes.

## CARRIER OILS

Apricot kernel oil: softening and soothing

Grapeseed oil: moisturizing and an antioxidant

Jojoba oil: an antioxidant, closely resembles natural sebum

Olive oil: moisturizing and an antioxidant

Sweet almond oil: soothing and anti-inflammatory

In this chapter, I use a very simple method for infusing your oils, known as the cold infusion method. There are also two other ways to infuse botanical oils and I have discussed these in detail on page 148, if you'd like to experiment with different methods.

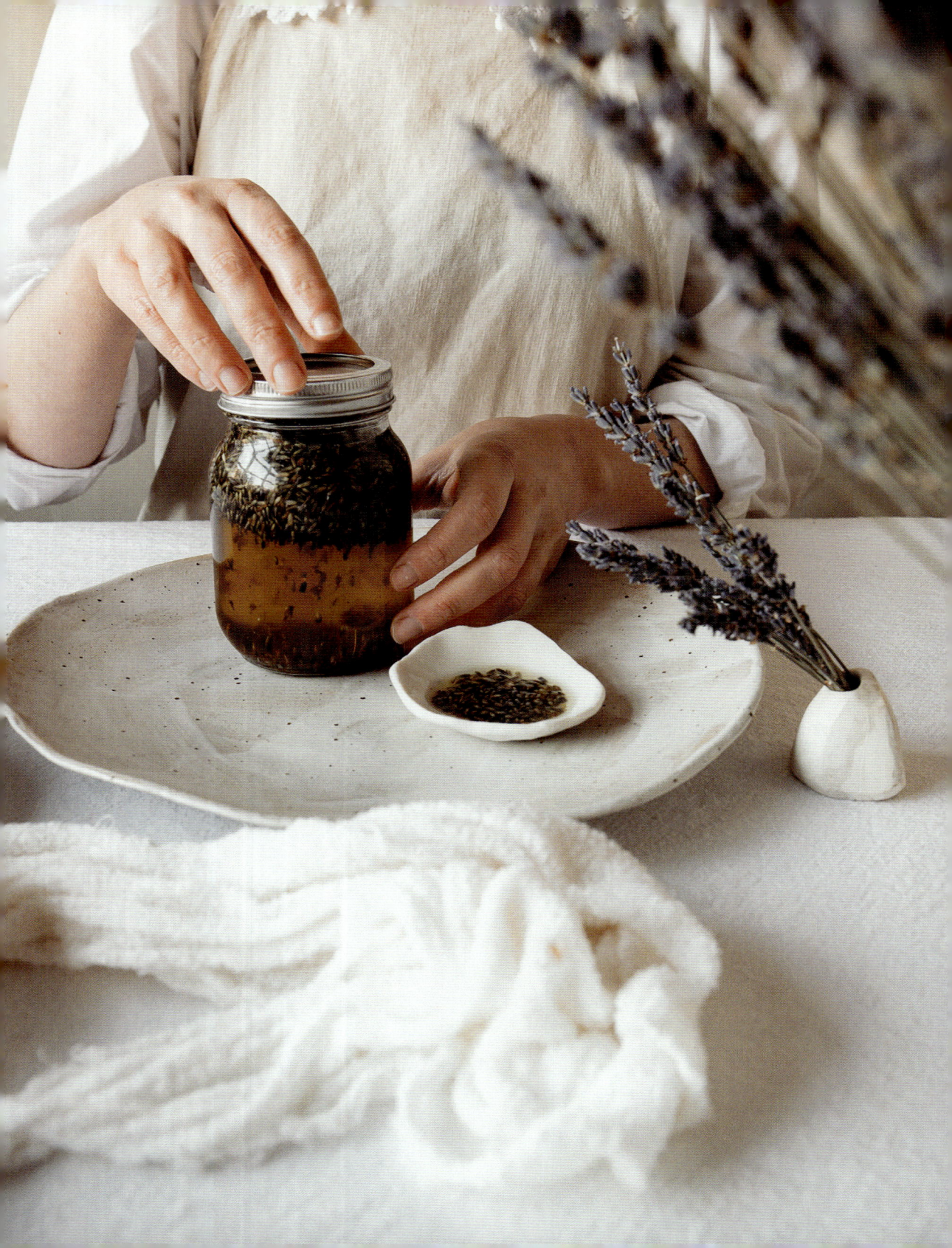

# LAVENDER INFUSED OIL

*Lavender is the most restorative fragrance for me. When I had my first child, the midwife who was caring for me advised me to add six drops to my bathwater with a cup of milk each night to help soothe my skin, prevent infections and relax me. Now, the smell of lavender transports me right back to that bubble of time, and I find it wonderfully calming and soothing, evoking the best memories.*

*Makes* 1 medium bottle (200 ml [¾ cup])

30 g (1 cup) dried lavender buds
250 g (1 cup) carrier oil

Loosely fill a medium-sized jar halfway with the lavender buds.

Pour your carrier oil over the lavender buds and fill the jar up to 1¼ centimeters (½ inch) from the top, then seal your jar with the lid.

Place the jar in a dark place at room temperature. A cupboard works well for this.

Allow the herbs to infuse in the oil for 4 weeks, turning occasionally.

Strain through a muslin cloth and store your infused oil in a clean, sterile bottle.

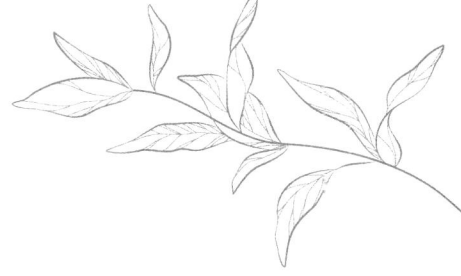

## Get to Know Your Ingredients!

When used in skin care, the lavender flower has natural anti-inflammatory properties, making it effective for soothing inflamed or irritated skin. It has been known to help treat skin problems such as eczema and psoriasis, and is also beneficial in treating acne flare-ups and helps to treat those blemishes in the skin.

The scent of lavender flower is well-known as being one of the best natural remedies to positively impact mood and mental well-being, as well as reducing stress. It can also help to promote better sleep and even treat headaches and pain.

# CALENDULA INFUSED OIL

*Calendula is another wonderful soothing botanical that can be used throughout your skin care recipes to heal and protect your skin. I love to grow calendula in my garden each year and harvest its golden petals to add sunshine to my recipes. It is a powerful but gentle botanical that is suitable for even the most sensitive skin.*

*Makes* 1 medium bottle (200 ml [¾ cup])

20 g (1 cup) dried calendula petals
250 g (1 cup) carrier oil

Loosely fill a medium-sized jar to the top with the calendula petals.

Pour your carrier oil over the calendula petals and fill the jar up to 1¼ centimeters (½ inch) from the top, then seal your jar with the lid.

Place the jar in a dark place at room temperature. A cupboard works well for this.

Allow the herbs to infuse in the oil for 4 weeks, turning occasionally.

Strain through a muslin cloth and store your infused oil in a clean, sterile bottle.

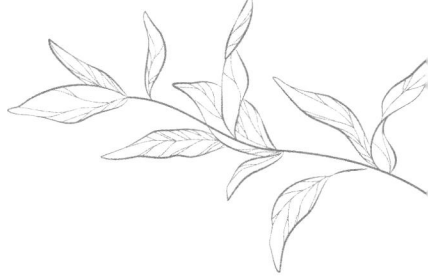

## Get to Know Your Ingredients!

Did you know that ancient Egyptians and Romans used calendula for cosmetic and medicinal purposes? It is valued as a wound-healing plant and thought to help regenerate skin cells and exert a calming and relaxing effect. Calendula contains high amounts of plant-based antioxidants that protect our skin cells from being damaged. It is a great ingredient for sunburns, acne and even rashes.

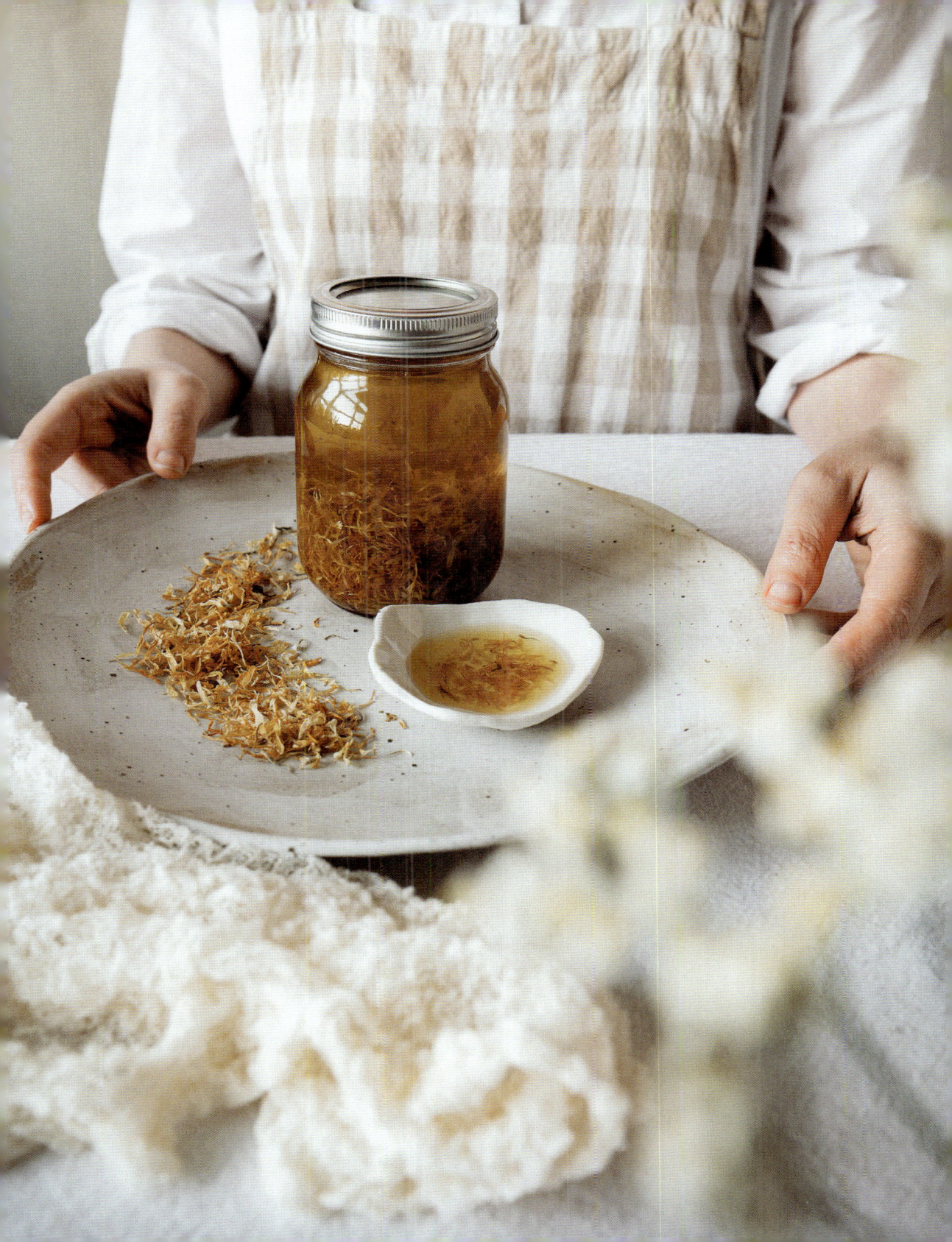

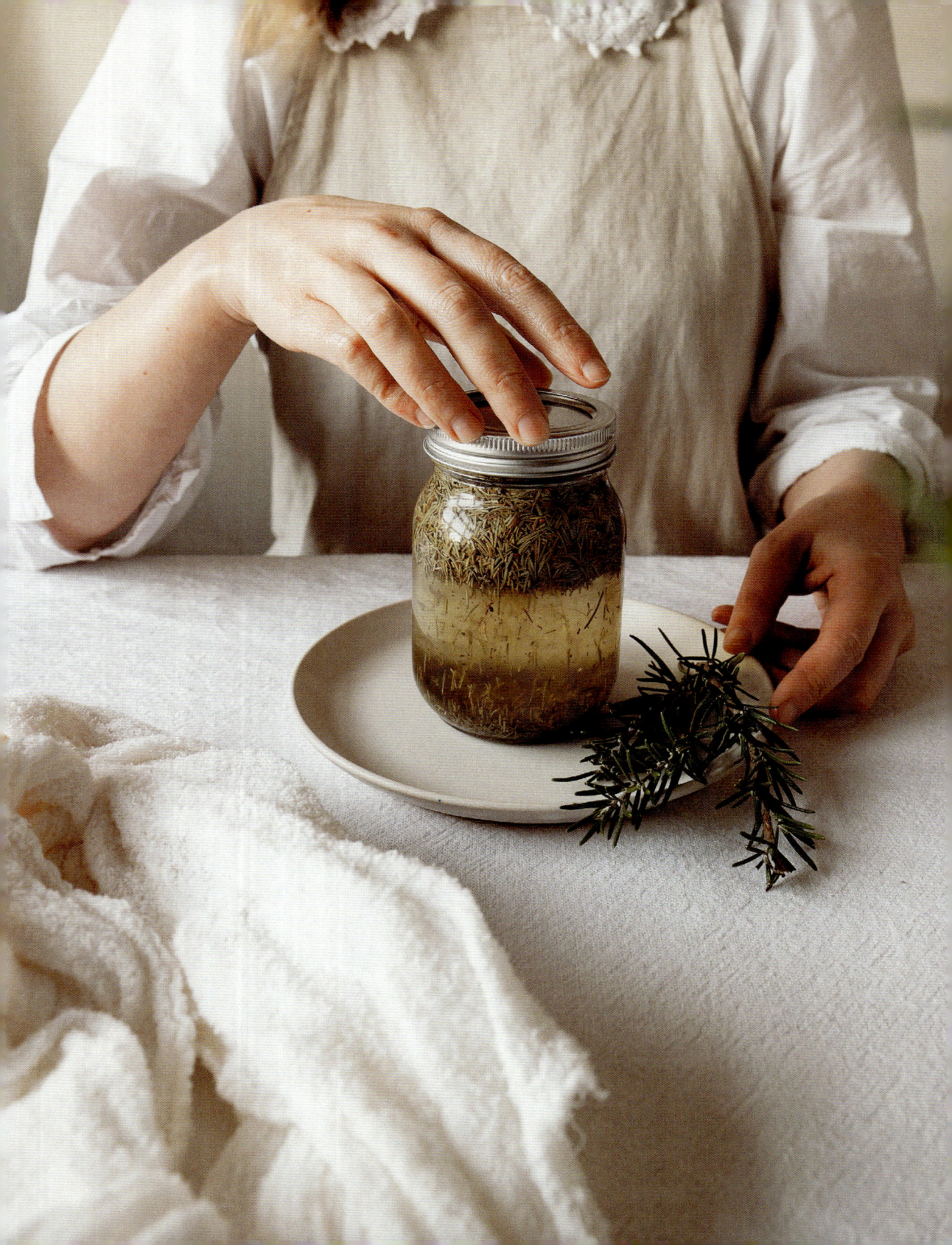

# ROSEMARY INFUSED OIL

*Rosemary is an herb that I just love to add to everything: skin care, hair care and my food! I also grow this herb in my garden, and whenever I walk past, I rub the leaves between by hands and inhale the aroma, as it helps to relax me and improve brain function and concentration!*

---

*Makes* 1 medium bottle (200 ml [¾ cup])

---

30 g (¾ cup) dried rosemary

250 g (1 cup) carrier oil

Loosely fill a medium-sized jar halfway with the rosemary. Pour carrier oil over the rosemary and fill the jar up to 1¼ centimeters (½ inch) from the top, then seal your jar with the lid.

Place the jar in a dark place at room temperature. A cupboard works well for this. Allow the herbs to infuse in the oil for 4 weeks, turning occasionally.

Strain through a muslin cloth and store your infused oil in a clean, sterile bottle.

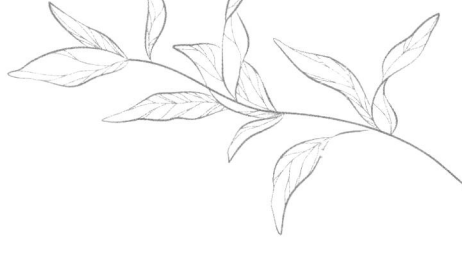

## Get to Know Your Ingredients!

Rosemary contains antioxidants that help to protect the skin from free radicals, reducing the risk of environmental damage and premature aging. When used in skin care, rosemary also helps balance oil production, which makes it a useful botanical for those with oily or acne-prone skin. Rosemary is also known to be restorative for hair and helps to promote hair growth and shine.

It is one of my favorite herbs to use throughout my home and it is also known to help lower cortisol levels and reduce anxiety.

# ROSE PETAL INFUSED OIL

*If you want glowing skin, look no further than rose petals. Roses are hydrating and illuminating for the skin, as well as adding the most wonderful fragrance to your skin care. As well as infusing dried rose petals in oil, you can add them into lots of your skin care ingredients. You will see that I have added them to face scrubs, bath oils and face masks in this book. You can also simply add them to your bathwater for a relaxing and restorative bath!*

Loosely fill a medium-sized jar to the top with the rose petals. Pour carrier oil over the rose petals and fill the jar up to 1¼ centimeters (½ inch) from the top, then seal your jar with the lid.

Place the jar in a dark place at room temperature. A cupboard works well for this. Allow the herbs to infuse in the oil for 4 weeks, turning occasionally.

Strain through a muslin cloth and store your infused oil in a clean, sterile bottle.

*Makes* 1 medium bottle (200 ml [¾ cup])

20 g (1 cup) dried rose petals
250 g (1 cup) carrier oil

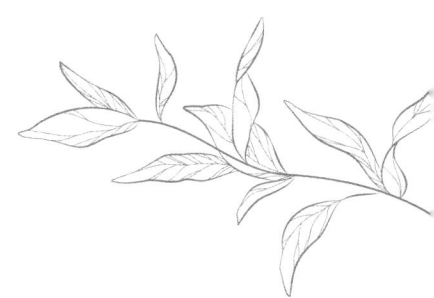

## Get to Know Your Ingredients!

Rose is well-known for its moisturizing and anti-aging properties. The antioxidants in rose petals can aid in preventing premature aging by reducing the appearance of fine lines, and they are a well-known ingredient used for hydrating and brightening your skin. The natural fragrance also promotes a calming and mood-enhancing effect.

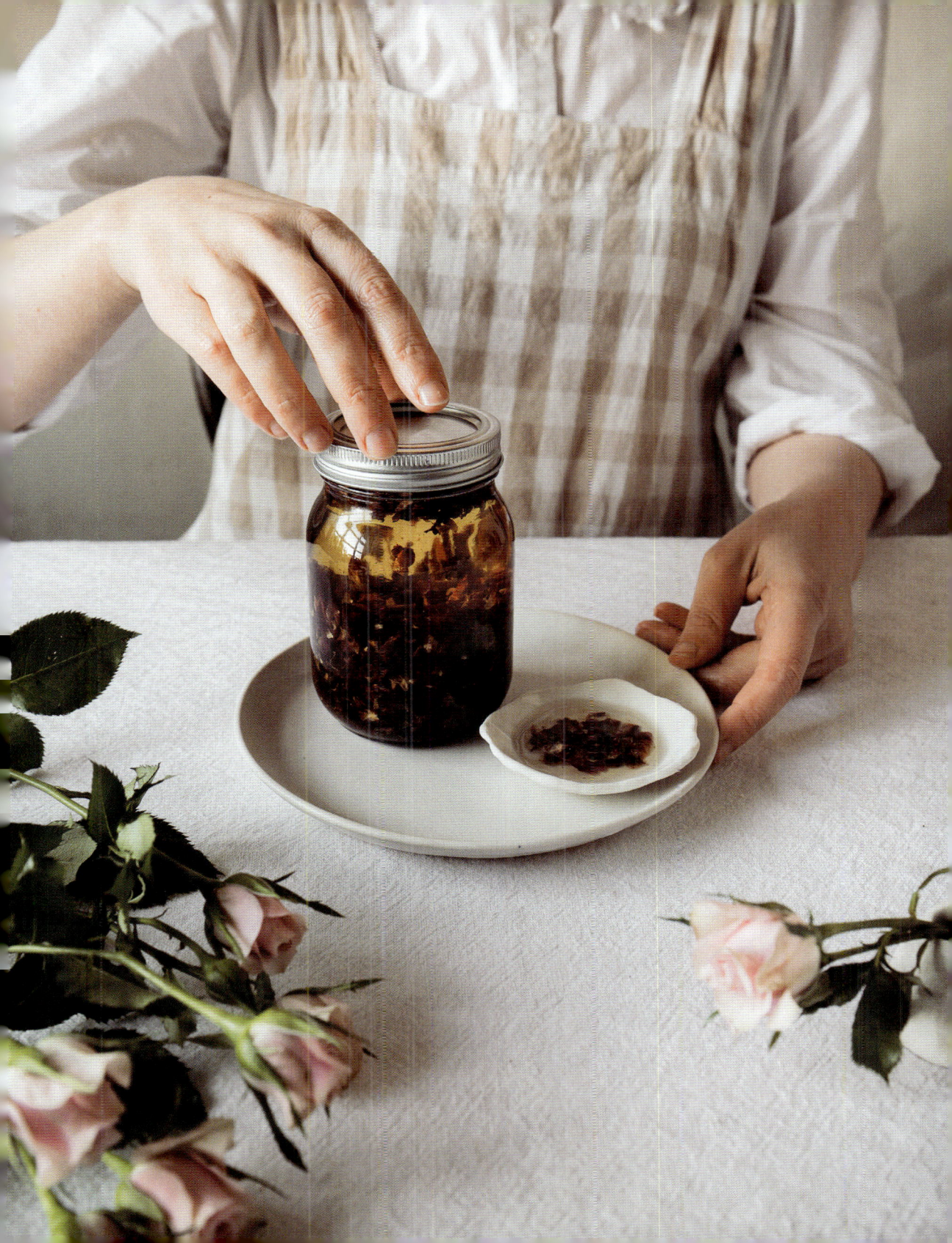

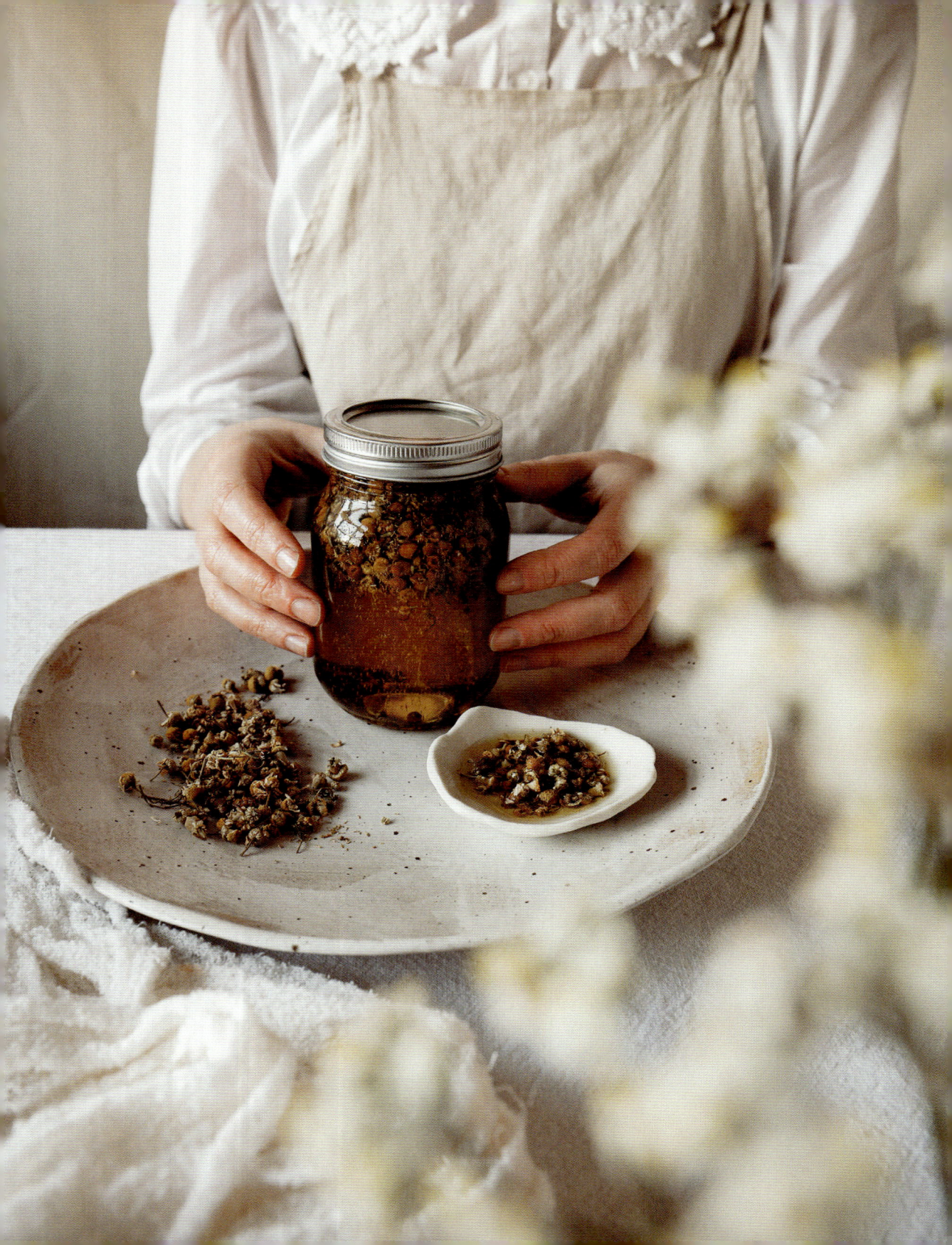

# CHAMOMILE FLOWER INFUSED OIL

*Did you know that the chamomile flower is considered a token of good luck? A gift of chamomile is seen as a wish of happiness and prosperity for its recipient, so share your chamomile recipes with your friends! As well as using chamomile in my skin care recipes, I also like to drink chamomile tea in the evening to help reduce stress and promote sleep.*

*Makes* 1 medium bottle (200 ml [¾ cup])

20 g (½ cup) chamomile flowers
250 g (1 cup) carrier oil

Loosely fill a medium-sized jar halfway with the chamomile flowers. Pour the carrier oil over the chamomile flowers and fill the jar up to 1¼ centimeters (½ inch) from the top, then seal your jar with the lid.

Place the jar in a dark place at room temperature. A cupboard works well for this. Allow the herbs to infuse in the oil for 4 weeks, turning occasionally.

Strain through a muslin cloth and store your infused oil in a clean sterile bottle.

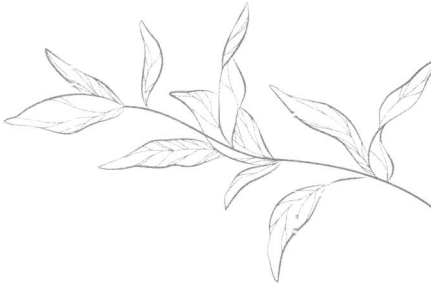

## Get to Know Your Ingredients!

Chamomile is well-known for its calming effects on the skin. It helps soothe irritation and redness and is suitable for sensitive skin. Chamomile has been traditionally used as a wound-healing ingredient and can help promote the regeneration of skin cells, which makes it a fantastic ingredient to include in your skin care recipes.

# ROSEHIP INFUSED OIL

*Rosehip oil has been used throughout history to treat infections such as coughs, colds, flu and respiratory conditions. When used in skin care, it is thought to protect your skin cells from damage and has long been used as a remedy for wound healing.*

*Makes* 1 medium bottle (200 ml [¾ cup])

30 g (¾ cup) dried rosehip
250 g (1 cup) carrier oil

Loosely fill a medium-sized jar halfway with the rosehip. Pour the carrier oil over the rosehip and fill the jar up to 1¼ centimeters (½ inch) from the top, then seal your jar with the lid.

Place the jar in a dark place at room temperature. A cupboard works well for this. Allow the herbs to infuse in the oil for 4 weeks, turning occasionally.

Strain through a muslin cloth and store your infused oil in a clean, sterile bottle.

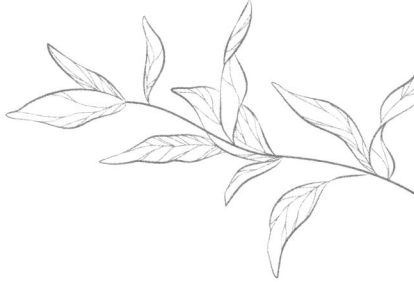

## Get to Know Your Ingredients!

Rosehips contain essential fatty acids that help moisturize and rejuvenate the skin. They are rich in vitamins and antioxidants, as well as having anti-inflammatory properties, which help soothe sensitive skin, hydrate the skin and improve moisture levels.

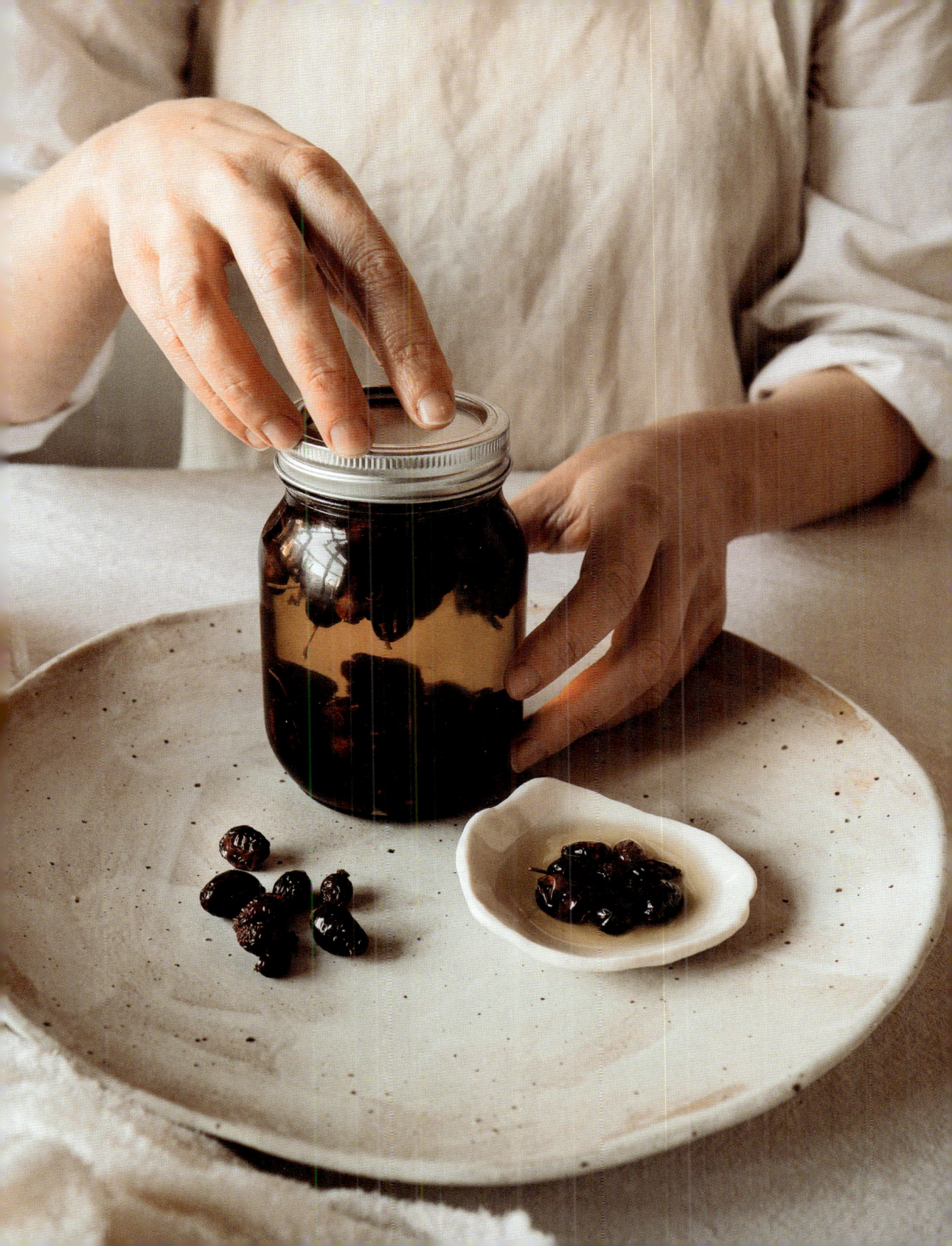

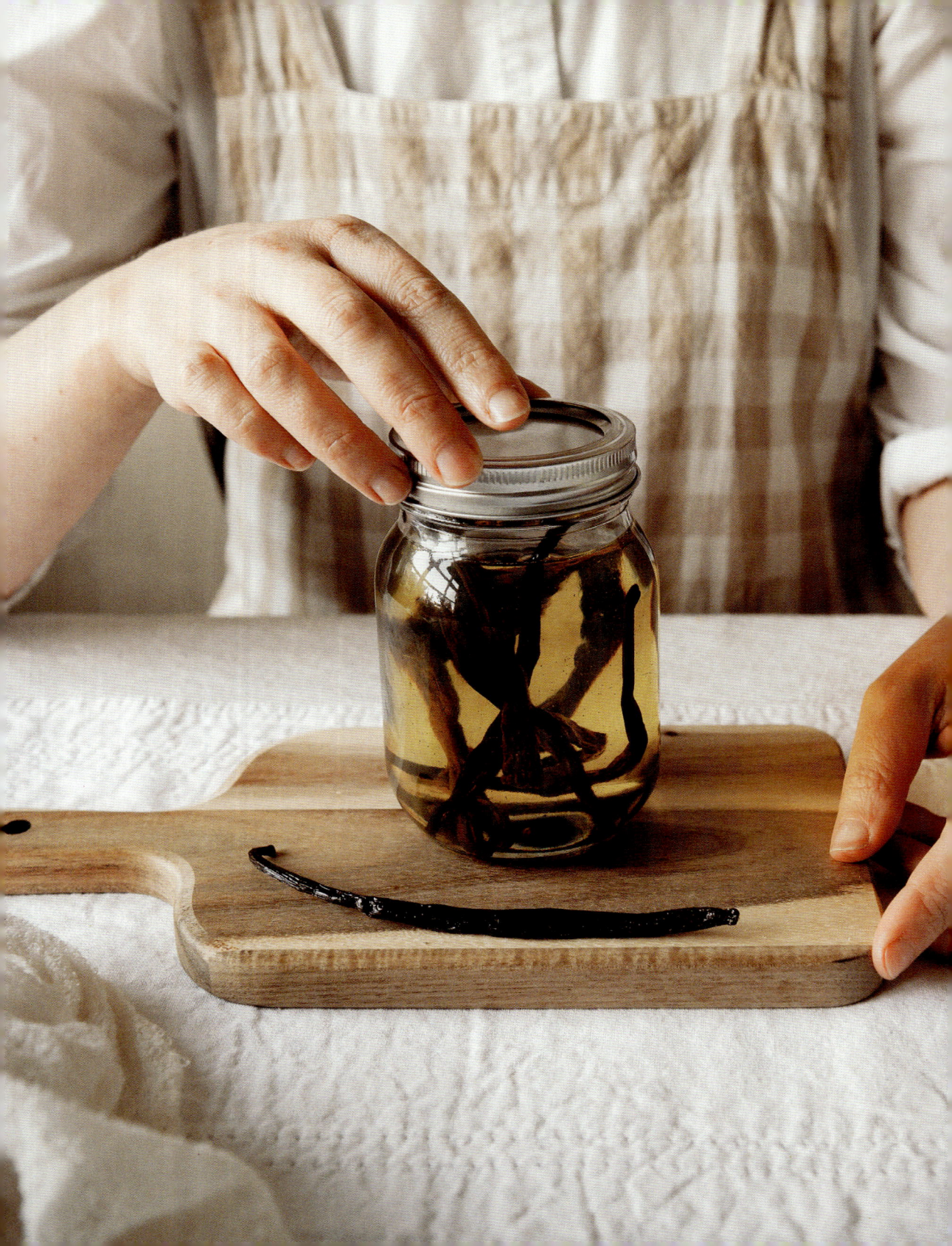

# VANILLA POD INFUSED OIL

*As you can imagine, this oil smells absolutely amazing! I use it in so many of my recipes to create a rich, delicious aroma, but in addition to this, it is also a good source of essential oils that help to protect your skin.*

*Makes* 1 medium bottle (200 ml [¾ cup])

4 vanilla pods
250 g (1 cup) carrier oil

Add your vanilla pods to your jar. Pour the carrier oil over them and fill the jar up to 1¼ centimeters (½ inch) from the top, then seal your jar with the lid.

Place the jar in a dark place at room temperature. A cupboard works well for this. Allow the vanilla pods to infuse in the oil for 4 weeks, turning occasionally.

Strain through a muslin cloth and store your infused oil in a clean, sterile bottle.

## Get to Know Your Ingredients!

Vanilla's rich scent creates a relaxing sensory experience when infused in oil. It is well-known in skin care for its beautiful fragrance, so it may surprise you that it also holds a number of protective properties for the skin. Vanilla contains B vitamins, contributing to healthy skin maintenance, and has antioxidants and soothing properties.

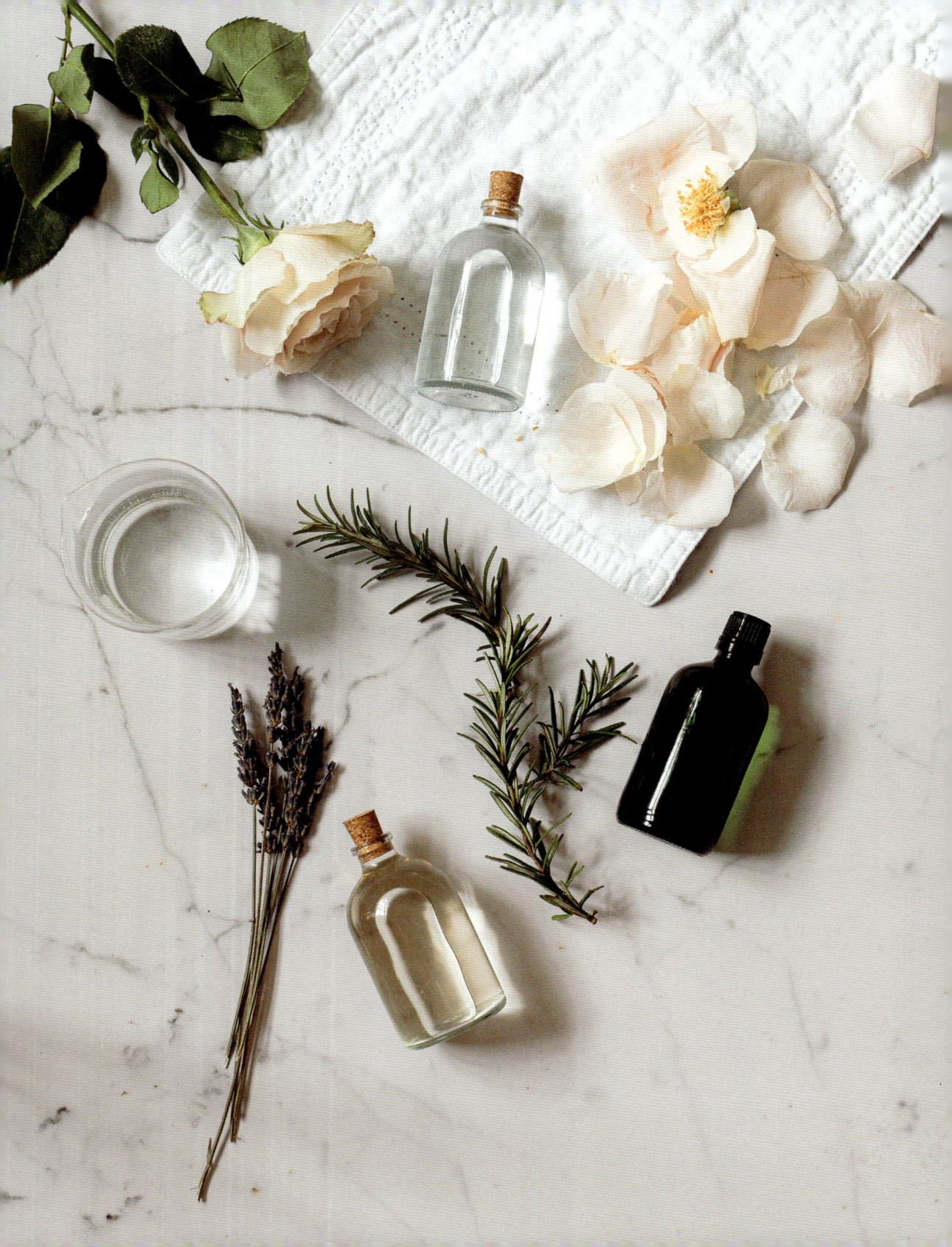

# BOTANICAL HYDROSOLS

Within the recipes of this guide, I often use botanical infused hydrosols. You can either buy these hydrosols ready made or you can make your own in the kitchen! It is worth noting that although I refer to these as hydrosols, they are not scientifically the same and are more of a botanical infused distilled water. They still smell amazing and are infused with the plant material, but a true hydrosol needs specific equipment that cannot be found in the kitchen. This version is a great alternative.

Hydrosols help to refresh and hydrate your skin, and can be used on even the most sensitive skin types. I love to use them in my cleansers to help remove every last impurity in my skin, and I also love to use them in my toners and face mists to help hydrate my skin and keep it supple throughout the day. They are also a welcome addition to my day bag during the hot summer weather when I use them as a face spritz to stay refreshed.

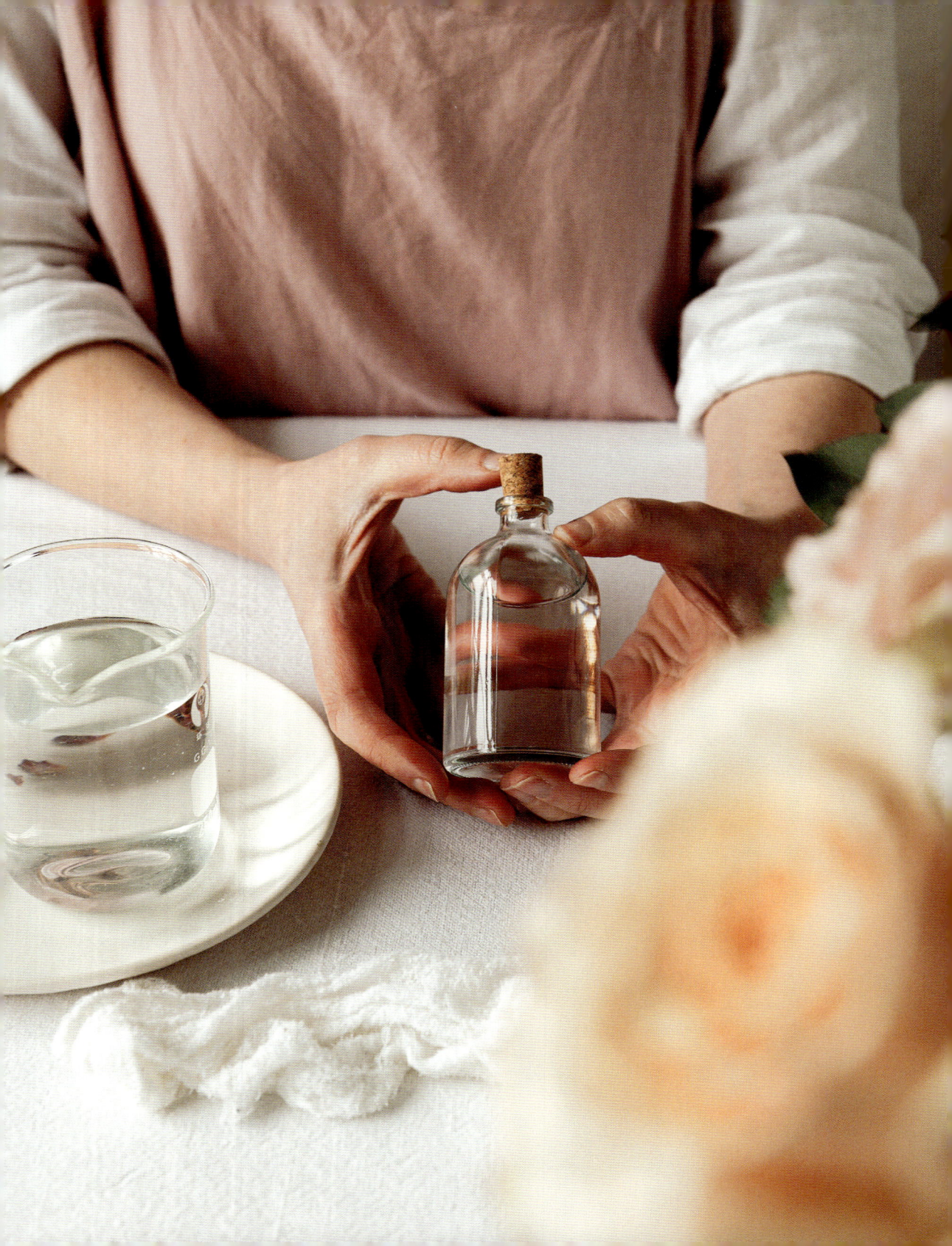

# DIY ROSE WATER HYDROSOL

*Rose petals are anti-inflammatory and contain antioxidants, which can help soothe the skin and reduce redness. Rose petals are also refreshing and rejuvenating for the skin.*

*Makes* 1 medium bottle (200 ml [¾ cup])

200 g (5 cups) rose petals
1 L (4½ cups) water

Add the rose petals (dried or fresh) and water to a large pan. Place a heat-resistant bowl in the center of the pan.

Heat your pan on medium heat and let the water boil. Place the lid of the pan upside-down over the pot and fill the top with ice. This will create condensation as the steam from the boiling water hits the ice-cold lid. The condensation will begin to drip into the bowl, leaving you with your botanical distilled water.

Allow to cool and transfer to a clean, sterile container.

This will need preserving. If you are using it straight away in one of the recipes, the preservative in the recipe will be adequate to use. If you are storing it to use later, it will only last up to 3 days in the fridge. A good way to store it if you are waiting to make a recipe with it would be to freeze the water until it is ready to be used. I like to freeze it into ice cubes, as it is easier to defrost a smaller amount to use rather than defrosting the full amount.

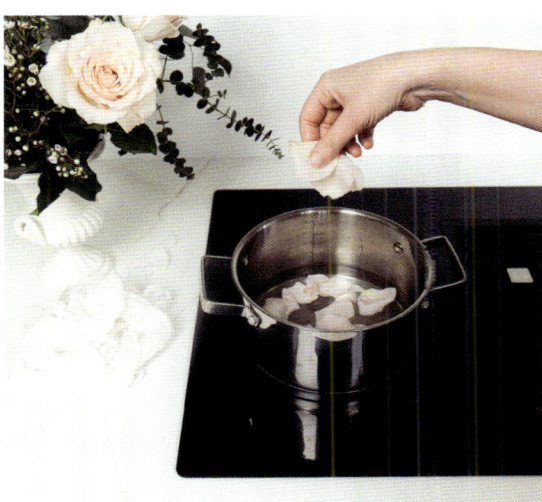

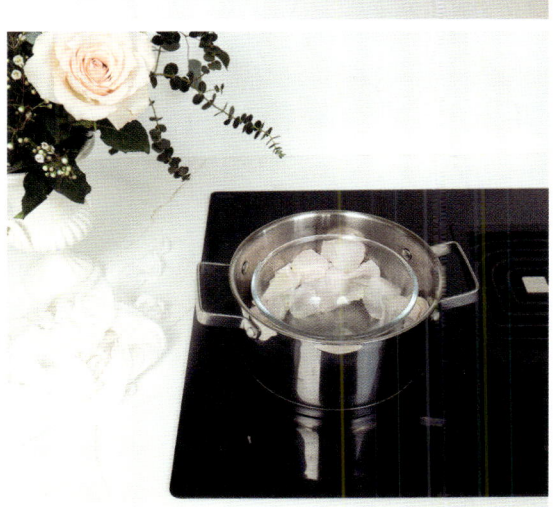

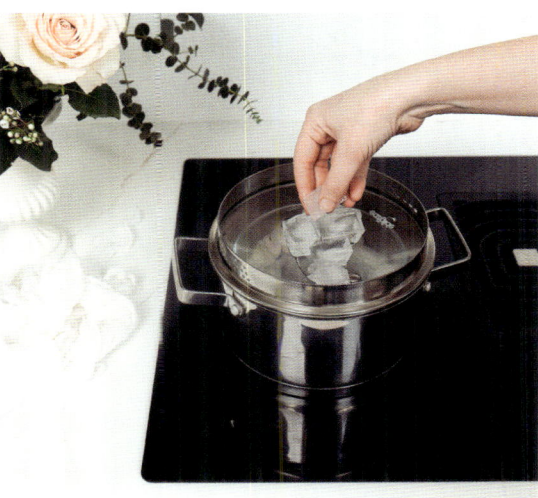

# DIY CHAMOMILE HYDROSOL

*The chamomile flower has many benefits when used in skin care and has anti-inflammatory and antioxidant properties. It is great for sensitive skin, as well as for soothing irritated skin, and can also reduce redness and promote healing.*

*Makes* 1 medium bottle (200 ml [¾ cup])

100 g (3½ cups) chamomile flowers
1 L (4½ cups) water

Add the chamomile flowers (either fresh or dried) and water to a large pot. Place a heat-resistant bowl in the center of the pot.

Heat your pot on medium heat and let the water boil. Place the lid of the pot upside-down over the pot and fill the top with ice. This will create condensation as the steam from the boiling water hits the ice-cold lid. The condensation will begin to drip into the bowl, leaving you with your botanical distilled water.

Allow to cool and transfer to a clean, sterile container.

This will need preserving. If you are using it straight away in one of the recipes, the preservative in the recipe will be adequate to use. If you are storing it to use later, it will only last up to 3 days in the fridge. A good way to store it if you are waiting to make a recipe with it would be to freeze the water until it is ready to be used. I like to freeze it into ice cubes, as it is easier to defrost a smaller amount to use rather than defrosting the full amount.

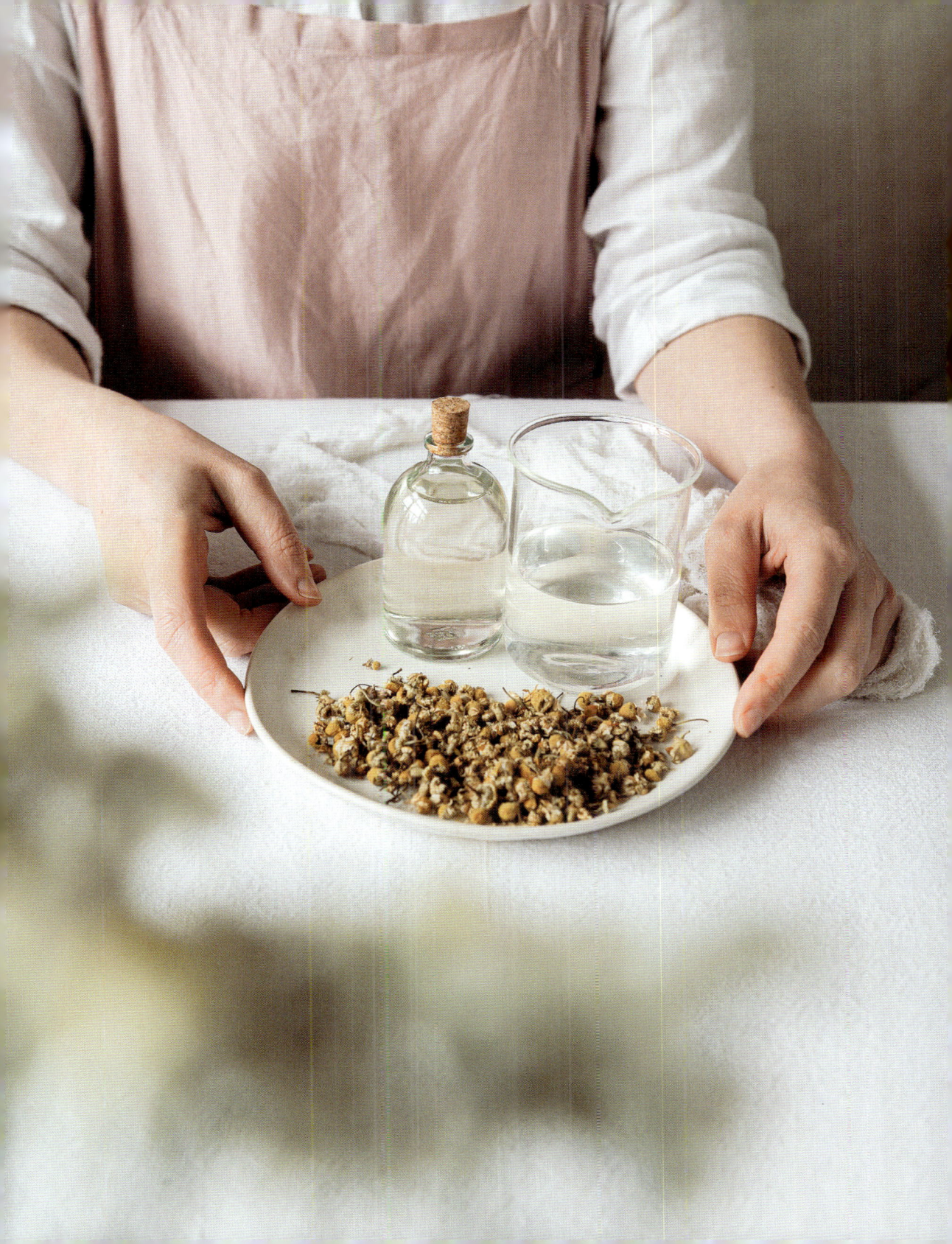

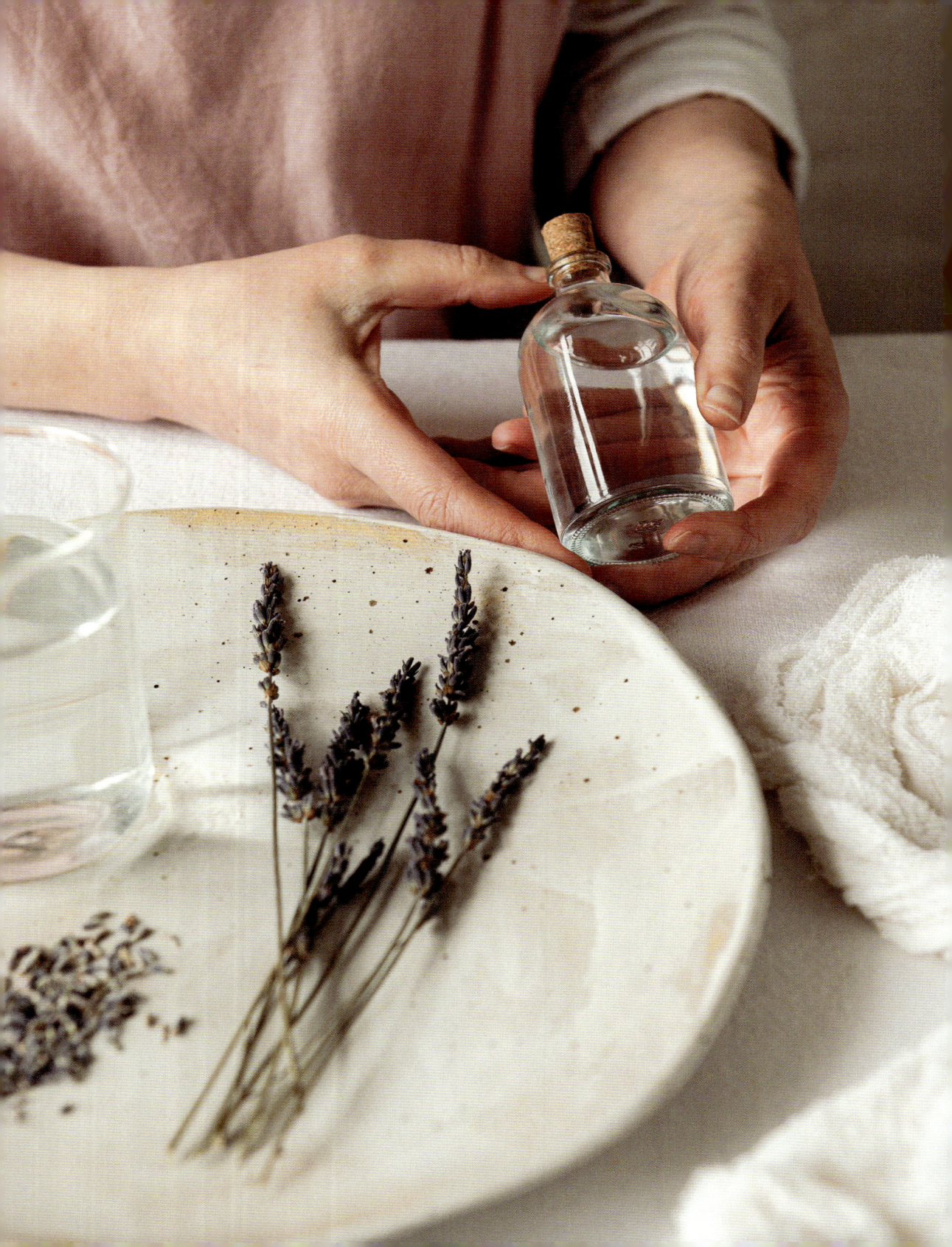

# DIY LAVENDER HYDROSOL

*The lavender flower is a beautiful addition to your skin care routine. Did you know that it has antibacterial and antifungal characteristics, which can aid in treating skin blemishes? The aroma of lavender is also known for its relaxation-inducing qualities, making it a great addition to your nighttime skin care routine.*

*Makes* 1 medium bottle (200 ml [¾ cup])

100 g (3 cups) lavender
1 L (4½ cups) water

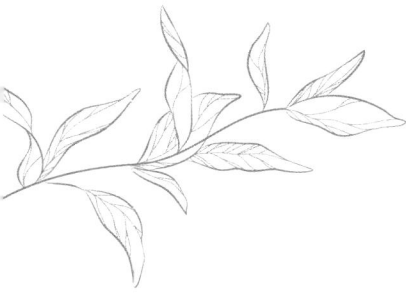

Add the lavender (either fresh or dried) and water to a large pan. Place a heat-resistant bowl in the center of the pan.

Heat your pan on medium heat and let the water boil. Place the lid of the pan upside-down over the pot and fill the top with ice. This will create condensation as the steam from the boiling water hits the ice-cold lid. The condensation will begin to drip into the bowl, leaving you with your botanical distilled water.

Allow to cool and transfer to a clean, sterile container.

This will need preserving. If you are using it straight away in one of the recipes, the preservative in the recipe will be adequate to use. If you are storing it to use later, it will only last up to 3 days in the fridge. A good way to store it if you are waiting to make a recipe with it would be to freeze the water until it is ready to be used. I like to freeze it into ice cubes, as it is easier to defrost a smaller amount to use rather than defrosting the full amount.

# DIY ROSEMARY HYDROSOL

*Rosemary has anti-inflammatory qualities, which help it calm and soothe irritated skin. It is commonly used in aromatherapy for its invigorating effects and is also thought to enhance mental clarity and focus.*

*Makes* 1 medium bottle (200 ml [¾ cup])

100 g (2¼ cups) rosemary
1 L (4½ cups) water

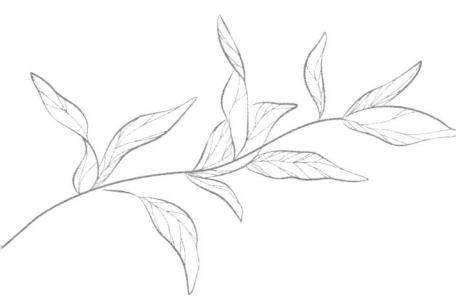

Add the rosemary (either fresh or dried) and water to a large pan. Place a heat-resistant bowl in the center of the pan.

Heat your pan on medium heat and let the water boil. Place the lid of the pan upside-down over the pot and fill the top with ice. This will create condensation as the steam from the boiling water hits the ice-cold lid. The condensation will begin to drip into the bowl, leaving you with your botanical distilled water.

Allow to cool and transfer to a clean, sterile container.

This will need preserving. If you are using it straight away in one of the recipes, the preservative in the recipe will be adequate to use. If you are storing it to use later, it will only last up to 3 days in the fridge. A good way to store it if you are waiting to make a recipe with it would be to freeze the water until it is ready to be used. I like to freeze it into ice cubes, as it is easier to defrost a smaller amount to use rather than defrosting the full amount.

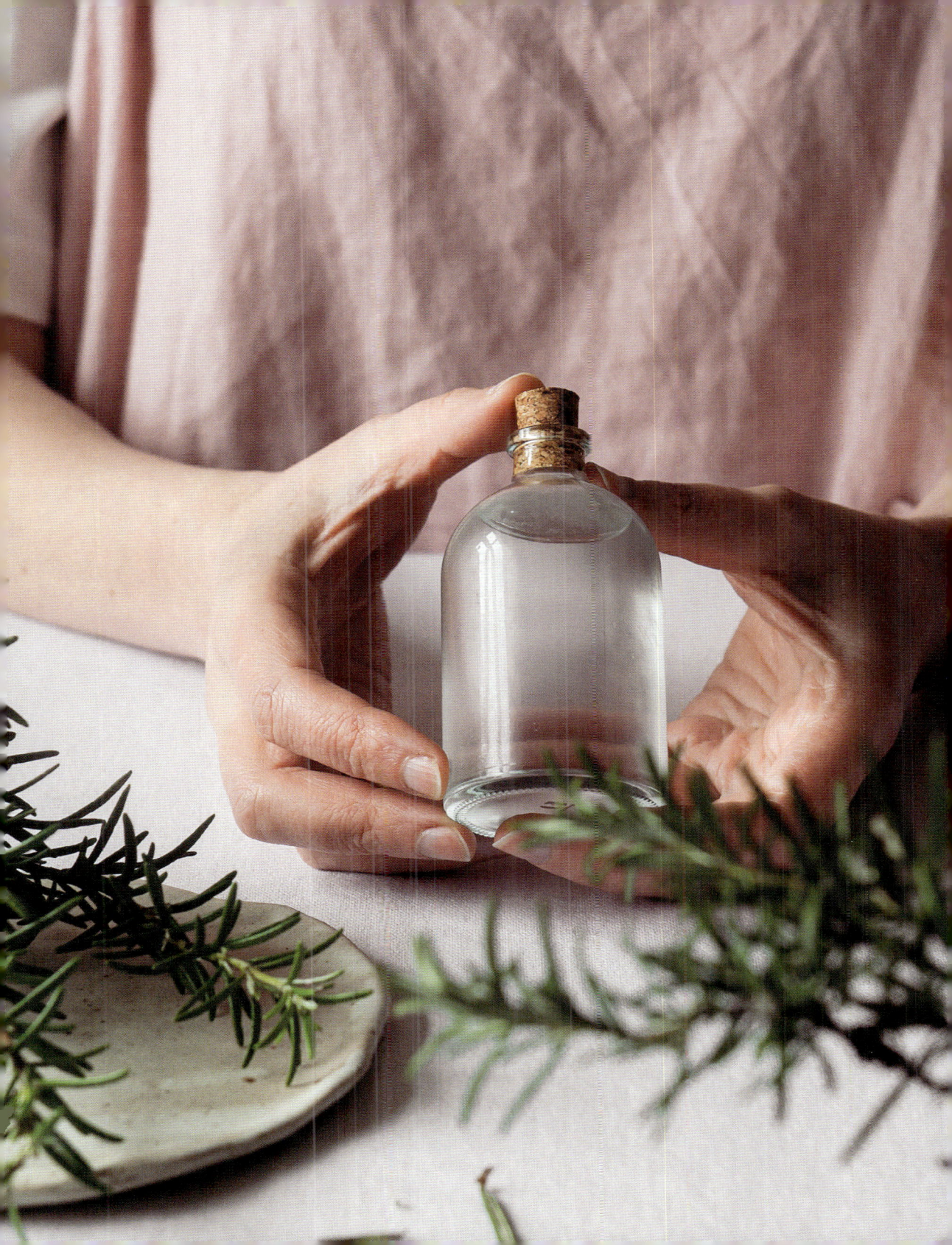

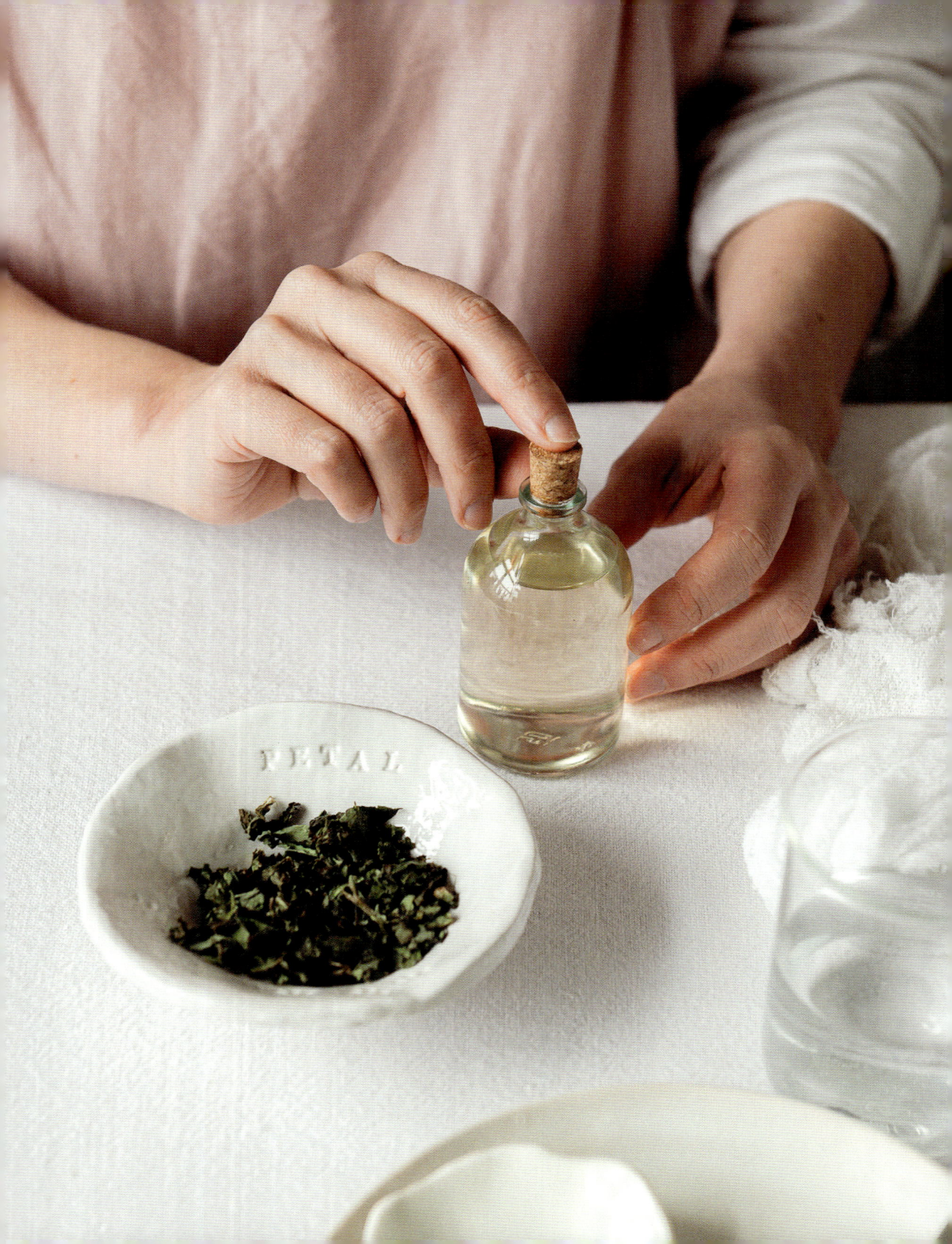

# DIY WITCH HAZEL HYDROSOL

*Witch hazel has anti-inflammatory properties, which help it calm redness and soothe irritated skin. It is also known as a natural astringent, helping to tighten and tone the skin.*

*Makes* 1 medium bottle (200 ml [¾ cup])

100 g (½ cup) witch hazel
1 L (4½ cups) water

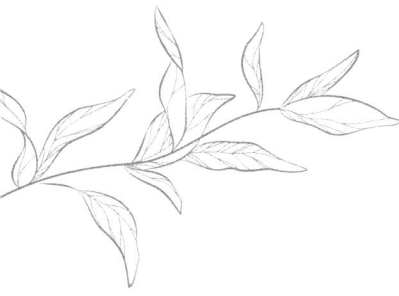

Add the witch hazel (either fresh or dried) and water to a large pan. Place a heat-resistant bowl in the center of the pan.

Heat your pan on medium heat and let the water boil. Place the lid of the pan upside-down over the pot and fill the top with ice. This will create condensation as the steam from the boiling water hits the ice-cold lid. The condensation will begin to drip into the bowl, leaving you with your botanical distilled water.

Allow to cool and transfer to a clean, sterile container.

This will need preserving. If you are using it straight away in one of the recipes, the preservative in the recipe will be adequate to use. If you are storing it to use later, it will only last up to 3 days in the fridge. A good way to store it if you are waiting to make a recipe with it would be to freeze the water until it is ready to be used. I like to freeze it into ice cubes, as it is easier to defrost a smaller amount to use rather than defrosting the full amount.

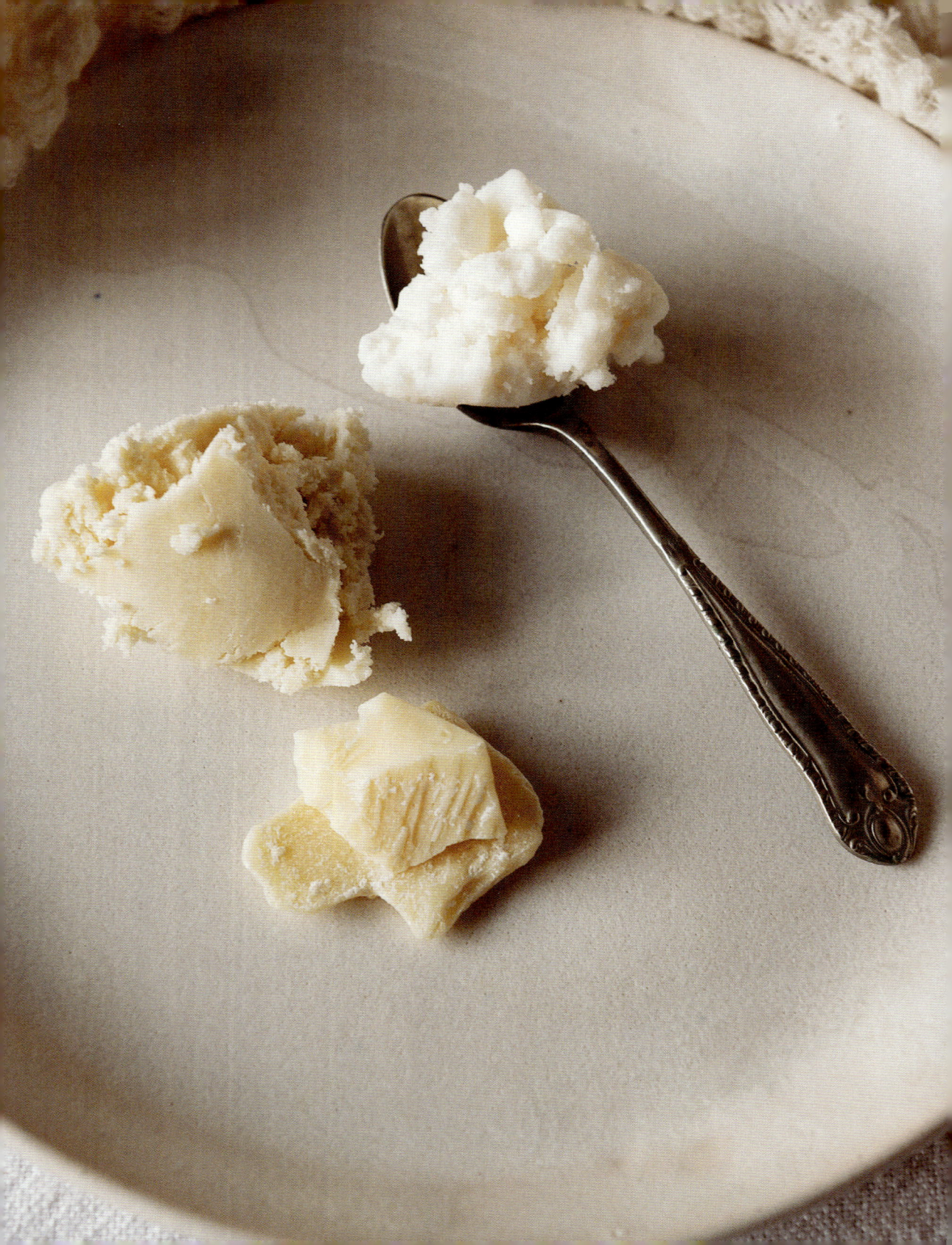

# METHODS AND GUIDES

If you are beginning your journey into natural skin care, there may be a few new methods within this book that you haven't seen before. Here, I have provided further information for you to learn more about them so that your skin care products are made exactly how you need them to be.

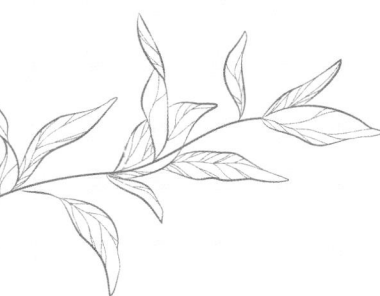

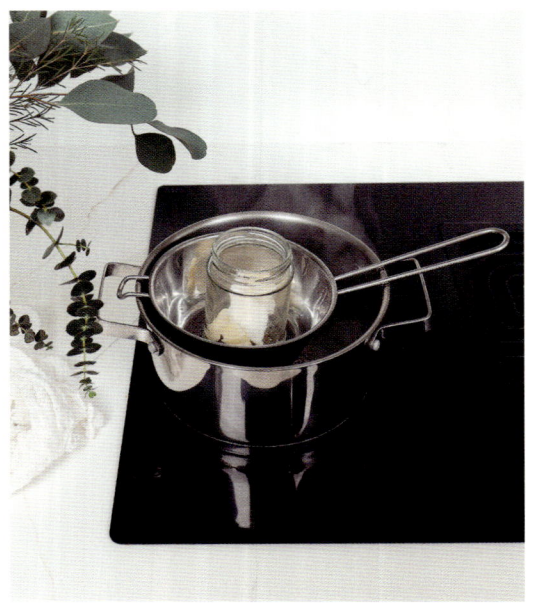

## THE DOUBLE BOILER METHOD

This is such a simple method to melt your butters and waxes until they are a liquid consistency and can be combined with your oils.

1. Using a pan, warm 2½ to 5 centimeters (1 to 2 inches) of water until simmering.

2. Place your heat-resistant bowl with your ingredients inside over the top. I use a small glass jar or Pyrex glass bowl. You want your bowl to fit snugly over the pan without touching the water.

3. Allow the water to gently simmer and melt the ingredient until it is liquid.

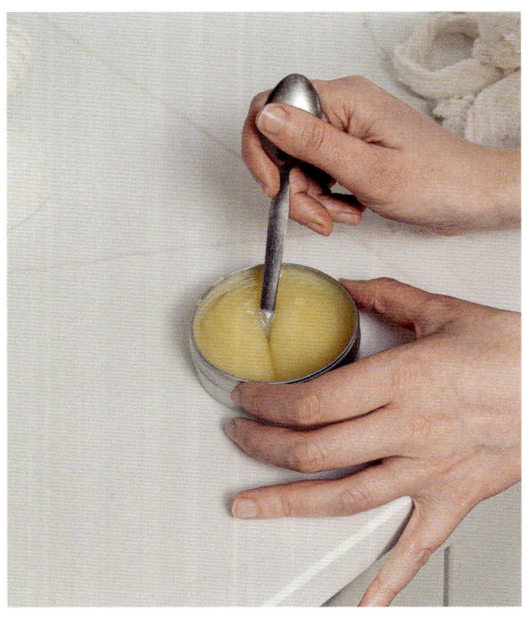

## FINDING A TRACE LINE

When you are making your own recipes in this book, I sometimes refer to finding a trace line. This can be done very easily and just requires a little patience. The reason that we need to find a trace line is that it ensures uniform distribution of ingredients, leading to product stability and effectiveness.

1. Make sure your ingredients are mixed together thoroughly.

2. Notice how the texture of your product changes from liquid to solid. This will take some time. Sometimes you will notice the color of the product change or sometimes you will notice the appearance of the product change as it starts to thicken.

3. As the mixture thickens, it will start to leave a very faint trail or "trace" when the tool you are mixing with is stirred through it. You can also perform a spoon test at this point and drip a very small amount of the mixture onto the recipe that you have made. If the droplet leaves a very faint mark on the surface before disappearing, you've found the trace.

# TROUBLESHOOTING BUTTERS AND BALMS

Here is a little step-by-step guide to managing any problems that may arise when you are creating your butters and balms.

### The recipe is too soft:

If your recipe is softer than you would like, you could try adding more hard butters to the recipe to make it firmer. You could modify your recipe by very gently melting it using the double boiler method (it will melt quickly on a low heat) and adding hard butter to the recipe, like cocoa butter. Repeat the remaining steps of the recipe to cool and create your lotion, butter or balm.

Another reason your recipe may feel softer than you would like could be due to living in a warmer climate. If so, you could either keep your recipe in the fridge (which would make it lovely and cooling when you apply it) or complete the step above to make it firm.

### The recipe is too hard:

If your recipe is harder than you would like, you could try adding a little extra oil to the recipe to soften it. You could modify your recipe by very gently melting it using the double boiler method (it will melt quickly on a low heat) and adding more carrier oil to the recipe, like sweet almond oil. Repeat the steps of the recipe to cool and create your lotion, butter or balm.

### The recipe is too grainy:

When using pure and natural ingredients like butters, there is always a possibility they may make your recipe grainy. You may have noticed this in natural products you bought from the shop before. It can happen after some time, and there isn't much we can do to prevent it. One thing to note is that it doesn't mean that there is something wrong with the recipe. It's still perfectly usable, although the touch and feel on the skin will not be the same.

You can easily fix this problem by very gently melting your recipe using the double boiler method (it will melt quickly on a low heat) and repeating the steps of the recipe to cool and create your lotion, butter or balm.

### The recipe smells unpleasant:

All the products that you create in this guide should be shelf-stable for up to six months. There are, however, variables, such as heat and oxidation, that could affect your recipes and reduce the shelf life. If this happens, you may notice that the recipe smells unpleasant and almost stale. This means that the product has turned rancid. If this happens, you should discontinue using the product.

# A GUIDE TO MAKING INFUSED OILS

There are three methods for infusing herbs into oil. I'm going to share all three of them so that you can choose which method you prefer.

## Cold Infusion Method

1. Sterilize a clean jar and ensure that it is dry.
2. Add your dried botanical to the jar.
3. Add your preferred carrier oil to your jar to completely immerse the botanical and fill your jar to the top, so that there is as little air as possible left in the jar.
4. Gently push your botanicals into the oil using a clean, sterile spoon to make sure you get rid of any air bubbles that may be remaining.
5. Place the lid on your jar and gently infuse for six weeks in a warm, dark place.
6. Turn the jars occasionally while the botanicals are infusing.
7. Strain the contents of the jar through a muslin cloth or similar. Gently squeeze to remove all the oil.

## Sun Infusion Method

1. Sterilize a clean jar and ensure that it is dry.
2. Add your dried botanical to the jar.
3. Add your preferred carrier oil to your jar to completely immerse the botanical and fill your jar to the top, so that there is as little air as possible left in the jar.
4. Gently push your botanicals into the oil using a clean, sterile spoon to make sure you get rid of any air bubbles that may be remaining.
5. Place the jar in a paper bag and put it on a sunny windowsill for six weeks to allow your botanicals to infuse.
6. Turn the jars occasionally while the botanicals are infusing.
7. Strain the contents of the jar through a muslin cloth or similar. Gently squeeze to remove all the oil.

## Heat Infusion Method

1. Sterilize a clean, heatproof mason jar and ensure that it is dry.
2. Add your dried botanical to the jar.
3. Add your preferred carrier oil to your jar to completely immerse the botanical and fill your jar to the top, so that there is as little air as possible left in the jar.
4. Gently push your botanicals into the oil using a clean, sterile spoon to make sure you get rid of any air bubbles that may be remaining.
5. Place your heatproof jar in a slow cooker with 5 centimeters (2 inches) of water surrounding it.
6. Do not put the lid on the slow cooker.
7. Gently heat over a very low heat (between 100 to 140°F [38 to 60°C]) for up to five hours, until the oil takes on the color and fragrance of the herb.
8. Strain your infused oil through a muslin cloth or similar. Gently squeeze to remove all the oil.

# A GUIDE TO STERILIZING JARS

When making your own skin care, it's important to add your products to clean, sterilized jars and vessels to ensure they last and stay fresh. Here is how I sterilize my jars in the oven. I also like to use isopropyl alcohol (70 percent) to keep my surfaces and utensils clean and sanitized when creating my recipes.

1. Heat your oven to 285°F (140°C).

2. Wash your jars and lids in warm soapy water. Next, rinse well to ensure no traces of soap are left. Do not dry your jars.

3. Place a piece of baking paper on a baking tray and place your wet jars on it, with the opening of the jar facing up. Ensure the jars aren't touching each other.

4. Place the jars in the oven for 20 minutes.

5. While the jars are in the oven, place your wet lids in a saucepan of water and boil for 20 minutes.

6. Take your lids out of the pan using clean tongs and dry thoroughly using a clean cloth.

7. Store in a clean area (a clean cupboard designated for your skin care products is a good idea) until they are ready to use.

# A GUIDE TO PRESERVATIVES

I use one antioxidant and one preservative throughout this skin care guide.

Vitamin E is commonly referred to as a natural preservative, but it is not actually a preservative. It is a powerful antioxidant that can extend the shelf life of waterless skin care products. Vitamin E has many beneficial properties, which is why I include it in the majority of my recipes, but one thing it can't do is prevent bacteria and mold growing in skin care products that contain water.

For this reason, I also use a preservative called preservative eco in all water-based recipes in this guide. Preservative eco is a broad-spectrum preservative that contains benzyl alcohol, salicylic acid, glycerine and sorbic acid. All of these ingredients can be extracted from natural sources, making this a natural preservative.

All products containing water or products that can easily be contaminated with water (e.g., sugar scrubs) need to have a preservative to make sure that they are safe for us to use. For bacteria and mold to grow in our skin care recipes, they need the presence of water, nutrients and oxygen—which will make our skin care products containing water the perfect hosts for this to happen. You absolutely do not want to be applying products to your delicate skin that may contain mold and bacteria.

Each recipe that I share will have instructions of how much preservative to add (when it is needed), and I encourage you to purchase a pair of jewelry scales that can measure 0.01 grams so that you can accurately measure the amounts needed.

# ESSENTIAL OIL INFORMATION

Essential oils are a beautiful way to boost your health and well-being in the form of aromatherapy. They have been used for centuries for both therapeutic and medicinal purposes and help to aid relaxation, boost your mood and improve your sleep, as well as reportedly being skin healing.

In recent years, however, essential oils have been debated a lot within green beauty circles. Firstly, the amount of plant material needed for a tiny bottle of essential oil is incredibly resource intensive. This is not as much of an issue if the plant material is readily available and the harvesting process is simple (e.g., lavender flower), but it is extremely damaging to our environment if the plant material is more resource intensive and over-harvested (e.g., frankincense).

The second issue is the toxicity of essential oils. Concerns have grown in recent years about whether these highly concentrated plant extracts are safe for common use. Simply put, if they are administered improperly, they can cause phototoxicity and dermal issues.

All of the recipes in this skin care guide have been crafted sympathetically to these issues. I have chosen to include only a small selection of ethically sourced essential oils, and I have taken care to ensure that the dermal limits of essential oils have been adhered to in every recipe. I feel that essential oils should be treated with the respect and care that they deserve while still being enjoyed within skin care products.

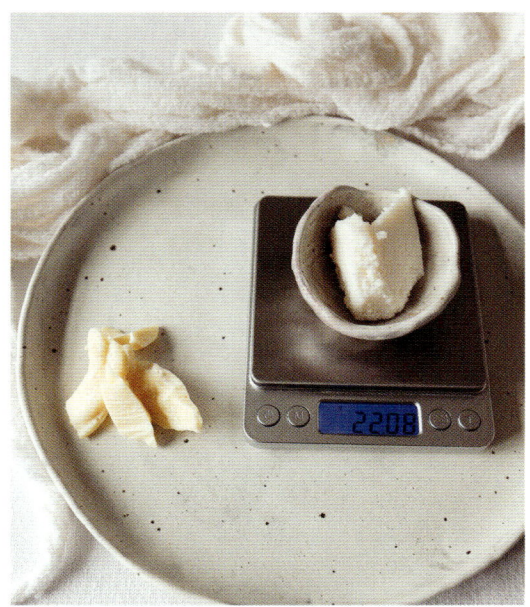

If you are pregnant, it is also important to conduct your own research regarding essential oils. Essential oils that should be avoided during pregnancy are clove, rosemary and clary sage, and I recommend not adding these to your recipes if you are pregnant.

I strongly recommend using a jewelry scale to measure your essential oils. In a pinch though, and if you are sure you are not sensitive to a specific type of essential oil, you can use the following ratio:

$$2 \text{ drops} = 0.2 \text{ g}$$
$$10 \text{ drops} = 0.5 \text{ g}$$

I am using a combination of essential oils and botanical infused oils in the recipes that I have included in this book, which will allow you to explore different ways to add botanicals and their fragrances to your products. It is entirely up to you if you choose to include the essential oils. My recipes will work beautifully with or without them.

## EQUIPMENT LIST

There's no need to buy lots of fancy equipment when you're making your own skin care recipes. I am providing a basic list of essential items, and you will likely find that you have the majority of these in your kitchen already.

Glass or stainless-steel bowl

Whisk, handheld

Spoons

Spatulas

Knife

Chopping board

0.01-gram jewelry scale

Hand blender

Large saucepan and lid

Medium-sized saucepan

Sieve to fit inside medium-sized saucepan

Heat-resistant bowl

Jars and lid or stainless-steel tins

Small glass bottles

Mini jars and lids or mini stainless-steel tins

Bottles and spray top

Labels

Silicone molds for lotion bars, toner bars, bath melts and bombs

70% isopropyl alcohol (rubbing alcohol) for disinfecting

## INGREDIENTS LIST

I've compiled all the ingredients used in this book in one easy list for you. You can refer to this when shopping. Make sure to read over the list carefully—you might already have a lot of this in your home.

**Carrier oils**
Apricot kernel oil
Castor oil
Coconut oil
Grapeseed oil
Jojoba oil
Olive oil
Sweet almond oil
Hemp seed oil
Rosehip oil

**Butters**
Mango butter
Shea butter
Cocoa butter

**Essential oils**
Bergamot
Geranium
Lavender
Mandarin
Peppermint
Rosemary
Chamomile
Clary sage
Rosehip
Clove
Tea tree

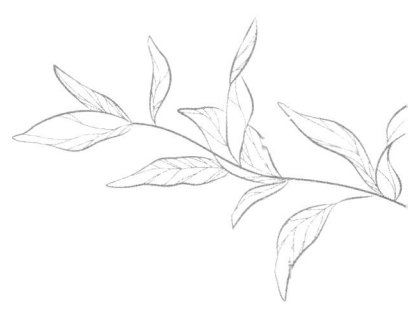

## Hydrosols
Rose water hydrosol
Lavender hydrosol
Witch hazel hydrosol
Chamomile hydrosol

*Remember that if you prefer, you can also make DIY hydrosols instead of buying these already made. See pages 133–143 for more information.*

## Botanicals
Bellis perrenis (daisy)
Calendula
Chamomile
Lavender
Rosehip
Rose petal
Rosemary
Vanilla pod
Witch hazel

*The botanical infused oils in this guide are interchangeable. When starting out, you could focus on creating two or three of these botanical infused oils and substituting them in the recipes that I have created for you.*

## Natural preservatives and antioxidants
Preservative eco
Vitamin E

## Waxes
Beeswax
Candelilla wax (vegan alternative to beeswax)

## Clays
Green clay
Kaolin clay
Rose kaolin clay

## Salts
Epsom salt

## Sugars
Caster sugar
Coconut sugar

## Additional ingredients
Adzuki beans
Baking soda (bicarbonate of soda)
Citric acid
Cornflour (cornstarch)
Liquid Castile soap
Oats
Vegetable glycerine

# SHELF STABILITY OF INGREDIENTS

All the ingredients in this book should be shelf-stable for up to six months. If the smell or appearance changes for the product, it may have been contaminated and I would recommend discontinuing its use.

If you would like to purchase a starter kit containing the ingredients listed in this book, you are able to at www.thenaturallivingshop.co.uk.

If you live in the United States, a good way to research your raw ingredients would be to look for soil association certified, organic and fair-trade products.

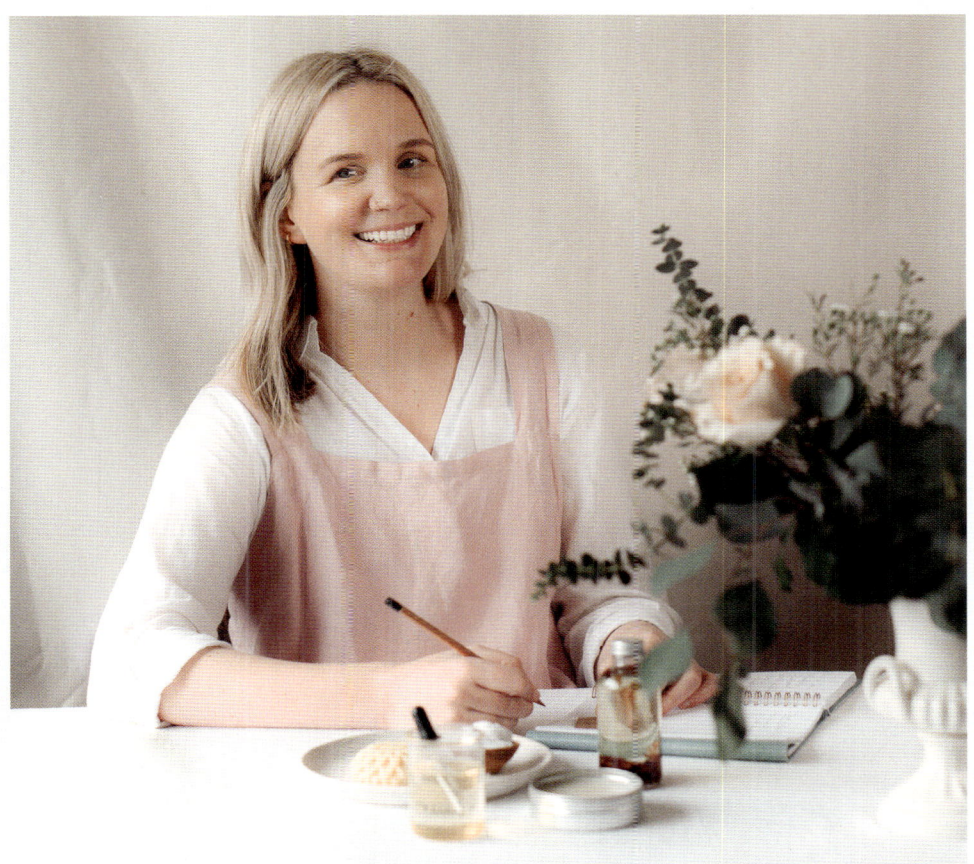

# ABOUT THE AUTHOR

Kate is a mum, a creator and the business owner of The Natural Living Shop, her eco-friendly refill shop. Kate runs her shop in her local community with the help of her husband, Michael, whose encouragement and support gave her the confidence and time to finally write this book. Kate loves to create and share sustainable living ideas online, and over the years, these ideas have helped others lead a more sustainable life too! Kate shares tutorials, recipes and advice on eco-conscious living on her popular Instagram page, My Plastic Free Home.

Her love for natural skin care stemmed from trying to find ways to find a nourishing, non-toxic skin care routine that was good her health and for the planet. She spent years paying money for skin care products that she now realizes were so overpriced and contained no real nourishment for her skin, leading to sensitivities and agitation. It was only when Kate embarked on this journey that she realized that less really is more. Through years of research and experimenting with beautiful butters, botanicals and oils, Kate is ready to share what she has learned with you all.

# ACKNOWLEDGMENTS

I could not have written this book without the support from my wonderful family. Thank you for believing that I can and encouraging me to be brave!

To my children, Etta and Roman: The way you love nature inspires me to explore and protect it in every way I can. You are my inspiration.

A little shout-out to the small businesses involved in writing this book:

https://thenaturallivingshop.co.uk/—My very own eco-friendly shop where you can find all of the natural ingredients for this book.

https://bohemiaphotos.com/—For Ale, my beautiful photographer, who showcased all of the ingredients in this book in the most beautiful way.

https://cheryltullyceramics.com/—For Cheryl, who allowed me to use all of her wonderful ceramics in the images. Your work is art Cheryl!

For Kate @oh.pea, my flowershop girl and other dreamy ceramicist. Thank you for lending me your lovely flower bowls.

https://www.cedarfarm.net/—The hub of so many small businesses (including mine!) and the heart of creativity for so many. Thank you for giving wings to my little ideas.

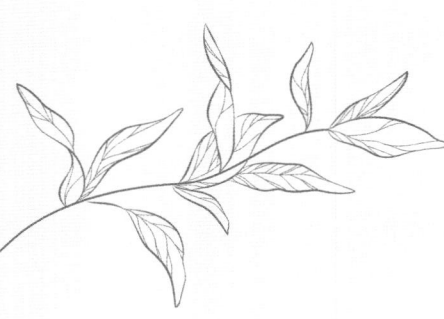

# MAKE YOUR OWN RECIPE!

# INDEX

Page numbers in **boldface** indicate illustrations.

## A
adzuki beans, 81
After-Sun Soothing Balm, **56**, 57
almond oil. *see* sweet almond oil
antioxidants, natural, 152
apricot kernel oil, 106, 117
Aromatherapy Massage Lotion Balm, **64**, 65

## B
baking soda, 101, 152
balms, 27, 55
    After-Sun Soothing Balm, **56**, 57
    Aromatherapy Massage Lotion Balm, **64**, 65
    Botanical Bruise Balm, 58, **59**
    Hydrating Lip Balm, **60**, 61
    Nourishing Cuticle Balm, 92, **93**
    Protective Balm, 34, **35**
    Repairing Lip Balm, 62, **63**
    troubleshooting, 147
bath bombs
    for children, 102
    Lovely Bubbles Bath Bombs, 102, **103**
    Relax and Unwind Bath Bombs, **100**, 101
bath indulgences, 95
bath melts
    Calming Bath Melts, **96**, 97
    Uplifting Bath Melts, 98, **99**
bath oils
    Botanical Bath and Body Oil, 106, **107**
    Soothing Bath and Body Oil, **104**, 105
bath salts
    Floral Bath Salts, 110, **111**
    Herbal Infused Bath Salts, **108**, 109
beeswax, 61, 92
bergamot essential oil, 97
body lotions and butters, 37
    Aromatherapy Massage Lotion Balm, **64**, 65
    Buttery Body Lotion, **42**, 43
    Calming Whipped Body Butter, 40, **41**
    Indulgent Whipped Body Butter, 44, **45**
    Nourishing Vitamin E Body Lotion, **38**, 39
body oils
    Botanical Bath and Body Oil, 106, **107**
    Soothing Bath and Body Oil, **104**, 105
body scrubs: Indulgent Sugar Body Scrub, **68**, 69
Botanical Bath and Body Oil, 106, **107**
Botanical Bruise Balm, 58, **59**
botanical hydrosols, 133
    DIY Chamomile Hydrosol, 136, **137**
    DIY Lavender Hydrosol, **138**, 139
    DIY Rose Water Hydrosol, **134**, 135
    DIY Rosemary Hydrosol, 140, **141**
    DIY Witch Hazel Hydrosol, **142**, 143
Botanical Micellar Cleansing Milk, 18, **19**
botanical oils, 117
    Calendula Infused Oil, 120, **121**
    Chamomile Flower Infused Oil, **126**, 127
    Lavender Infused Oil, **118**, 119
    Rose Petal Infused Oil, 124, **125**
    Rosehip Infused Oil, 128, **129**
    Rosemary Infused Oil, **122**, 123
    Vanilla Pod Infused Oil, **130**, 131
botanicals, 22, 98, 110
butters and balms, 151
    Get the Glow Cleansing Butter, **12**, 13
    troubleshooting, 147
Buttery Body Lotion, **42**, 43

## C
calendula, 44, 57, 120
Calendula Infused Oil, 120, **121**
    After-Sun Soothing Balm, **56**, 57
    Calming Bath Melts, **96**, 97
    Glow Face Oil, **28**, 29
    Indulgent Whipped Body Butter, 44, **45**
    Nourishing Cuticle Balm, 92, **93**

Calm and Tone Chamomile Sphere, **24,** 25
Calming Bath Melts, **96,** 97
Calming Oat Face Mask, 82, **83**
Calming Whipped Body Butter, 40, **41**
candelilla wax, 34, 152
carrier oils, 117, 151
caster sugar scrubs, 70
castor oil, 13, 87
chamomile, 57, 127
Chamomile Flower Infused Oil, **126,** 127
   Botanical Bruise Balm, 58, **59**
   Protective Balm, 34, **35**
Chamomile Hydrosol
   Calm and Tone Chamomile Sphere, **24,** 25
   DIY Chamomile Hydrosol, 136, **137**
children: bath bombs for, 102
clary sage essential oil, 114
clays, 152
cleansers, 11
   Botanical Micellar Cleansing Milk, 18, **19**
   Get the Glow Cleansing Butter, **12,** 13
   Nourishing Jojoba and Rose Bi-Phase Cleanser, **16,** 17
   Relax and Restore Creamy Cleanser, 14, **15**
clove essential oil, 65
cocoa butter, 49, 92, 97
coconut oil, 101
Cold Infusion Method, 148
common daisy (bellis perennis), 58
cornflour (cornstarch), 101
cuticle balms: Nourishing Cuticle Balm, 92, **93**

## D

daisy (bellis perennis), 58
Daisy Infused Oil: Botanical Bruise Balm, 58, **59**
Deep Muscle Massaging Bar, **48,** 49
DIY Chamomile Hydrosol, 136, **137**
DIY Lavender Hydrosol, **138,** 139
DIY Rose Water Hydrosol, **134,** 135
DIY Rosemary Hydrosol, 140, **141**
DIY Witch Hazel Hydrosol, **142,** 143
Double Boiler Method, 146, **146**

## E

Epsom salts, 101, 102, 109, 110, 113, 114
equipment, 151
essential oils, 15, 150–51
   adding, 9
   measurement ratios, 150
eucalyptus essential oil, 53
Everyday Rituals Massaging Lotion Bar, **52,** 53
Eyebrow Growth Oil, **90,** 91

## F

face masks, 75
   Calming Oat Face Mask, 82, **83**
   Green Clay Deep Cleanse Face Mask, 78, **79**
   Kaolin Caring Clay Mask, **80,** 81
   Rose Clay Hydrating Face Mask, **76,** 77
face oils, lotions and balms, 27
   Glow Face Oil, **28,** 29
   Nourishing Jojoba Face Lotion, **32,** 33
   Relax and Restore Facial Oil, 30, **31**
face scrubs: Glowing Face Polish, 70, **71**
face spritz: Relaxing Lavender Toner and Face Spritz, **20,** 21
Floral Bath Salts, 110, **111**

## G

Get the Glow Cleansing Butter, **12,** 13
Glow Face Oil, **28,** 29
Glowing Face Polish, 70, **71**
grapeseed oil, 105, 117
green clay, 78
Green Clay Deep Cleanse Face Mask, 78, **79**

## H

Hair Growth Oil, **86,** 87
Heat Infusion Method, 148
hemp seed oil: Relax and Restore Facial Oil, 30, **31**
Herbal Infused Bath Salts, **108,** 109
Hydrating Lip Balm, **60,** 61
Hydrating Rose Water Toning Bar, 22, **23**
hydrosols, 131, 152
   DIY Chamomile Hydrosol, 136, **137**
   DIY Lavender Hydrosol, **138,** 139

157

DIY Rose Water Hydrosol, **134**, 135
DIY Rosemary Hydrosol, 140, **141**
DIY Witch Hazel Hydrosol, **142**, 143

## I
Indulgent Sugar Body Scrub, **68**, 69
Indulgent Whipped Body Butter, 44, **45**
infused oils, 148, 152
ingredients, 151–52

## J
jojoba oil, 17, 117
    Nourishing Jojoba and Rose Bi-Phase Cleanser, **16**, 17
    Nourishing Jojoba Face Lotion, **32**, 33

## K
Kaolin Caring Clay Mask, **80**, 81
kaolin clay, 81–82, 110

## L
lavender, 40
lavender essential oil, 65, 97, 114
lavender flower, 119
Lavender Hydrosol, **138**, 139
    Botanical Micellar Cleansing Milk, 18, **19**
    Relaxing Lavender Toner and Face Spritz, **20**, 21

Lavender Infused Oil, 15, **118**, 119
    Botanical Bath and Body Oil, 106, **107**
    Calming Whipped Body Butter, 40, **41**
    Nourishing Jojoba Face Lotion, **32**, 33
    Relax and Restore Creamy Cleanser, 14, **15**
    Soothe Your Skin Massage Oil, 88, **89**
lip balms
    Hydrating Lip Balm, **60**, 61
    Repairing Lip Balm, 62, **63**
lip scrubs: Plumping Peppermint and Vanilla Lip Scrub, **72**, 73
lotion bars, 47
    Deep Muscle Massaging Bar, 48, 49
    Everyday Rituals Massaging Lotion Bar, **52**, 53
    Relaxing Massage Lotion Bar, 50, **51**
lotions, 27. *see also* body lotions and butters; face oils, lotions, and balms
Lovely Bubbles Bath Bombs, 102, **103**

## M
mandarin essential oil, 49, 113
massage bars, 47
    Deep Muscle Massaging Bar, 48, 49
    Everyday Rituals Massaging Lotion Bar, **52**, 53
    Relaxing Massage Lotion Bar, 50, **51**
massage lotion balms: Aromatherapy Massage Lotion Balm, **64**, 65
massage oils: Soothe Your Skin Massage Oil, 88, **89**
metric measurements, 9
micellar waters: Botanical Micellar Cleansing Milk, 18, **19**

## N
natural preservatives and antioxidants, 152
Nourishing Cuticle Balm, 92, **93**
Nourishing Jojoba and Rose Bi-Phase Cleanser, **16**, 17
Nourishing Jojoba Face Lotion, **32**, 33
Nourishing Vitamin E Body Lotion, **38**, 39

## O
oats: Calming Oat Face Mask, 82, **83**
olive oil, 88, 117

## P
peppermint essential oil, 13, 87, 113
Plumping Peppermint and Vanilla Lip Scrub, **72**, 73
precautions, 9
preservative eco, 149
preservatives, 149
    eco-friendly, 17
    natural, 152
Protective Balm, 34, **35**

## R

Relax and Restore Creamy Cleanser, 14, **15**
Relax and Restore Facial Oil, 30, **31**
Relax and Unwind Bath Bombs, **100**, 101
Relaxing Lavender Toner and Face Spritz, **20**, 21
Relaxing Massage Lotion Bar, 50, **51**
Repairing Lip Balm, 62, **63**
rose, 124
Rose Clay Hydrating Face Mask, **76**, 77
rose kaolin clay, 77
Rose Petal Infused Oil, 124, **125**
    Buttery Body Lotion, **42**, 43
rose petals, 124
rose water, 21–22
    Hydrating Rose Water Toning Bar, 22, **23**
    Nourishing Jojoba and Rose Bi-Phase Cleanser, **16**, 17
Rose Water Hydrosol, 17
    Botanical Micellar Cleansing Milk, 18, **19**
    DIY Rose Water Hydrosol, **134**, 135
    Hydrating Rose Water Toning Bar, 22, **23**
    Nourishing Jojoba and Rose Bi-Phase Cleanser, **16**, 17
Rosehip Infused Oil, 128, **129**
    Botanical Bath and Body Oil, 106, **107**
    Relax and Restore Facial Oil, 30, **31**
    Uplifting Bath Melts, 98, **99**
rosehip oil, 29
rosehips, 128
rosemary, 87, 91, 123
rosemary essential oil, 114
Rosemary Hydrosol, 140, **141**
Rosemary Infused Oil, **122**, 123
    Eyebrow Growth Oil, **90**, 91
    Hair Growth Oil, **86**, 87

## S

salts, 152
scrubs, 67
    caster sugar, 70
    Glowing Face Polish, **70**, 71
    Indulgent Sugar Body Scrub, **68**, 69
    Plumping Peppermint and Vanilla Lip Scrub, **72**, 73
    sugar, 149
shea butter, 50, 57
shelf stability, 152
shower steamers
    Sleepy Time Shower Steamers, 114, **115**
    Wake Up Shower Steamers, **112**, 113
silicone molds, 47
Sleepy Time Shower Steamers, 114, **115**
Soothe Your Skin Massage Oil, 88, **89**
Soothing Bath and Body Oil, **104**, 105
spritz: Relaxing Lavender Toner and Face Spritz, **20**, 21
sterilizing jars, 149
sugar scrubs, 149
sugars, 152
Sun Infusion Method, 148
sweet almond oil, 15, 40, 117

## T

tea tree essential oil, 113
testing products, 9
toners, 11
    Calm and Tone Chamomile Sphere, **24**, 25
    Hydrating Rose Water Toning Bar, 22, **23**
    Relaxing Lavender Toner and Face Spritz, **20**, 21
trace lines, **146**, 146–47
treatment oils, 85
    Eyebrow Growth Oil, **90**, 91
    Hair Growth Oil, **86**, 87
    Nourishing Cuticle Balm, 92, **93**
    Soothe Your Skin Massage Oil, 88, **89**
    Soothing Bath and Body Oil, **104**, 105
troubleshooting butters and balms, 147

## U
Uplifting Bath Melts, 98, **99**

## V
vanilla, 131
Vanilla Pod Infused Oil, **130**, 131
    Calming Whipped Body Butter, 40, **41**
    Get the Glow Cleansing Butter, **12**, 13
    Indulgent Sugar Body Scrub, **68**, 69
    Nourishing Jojoba Face Lotion, **32**, 33
    Plumping Peppermint and Vanilla Lip Scrub, **72**, 73
    Soothe Your Skin Massage Oil, 88, **89**
vanilla pods, 105
vitamin E, 149
    Nourishing Vitamin E Body Lotion, **38**, 39

## W
Wake Up Shower Steamers, **112**, 113
waxes, 152
witch hazel, 21
Witch Hazel Hydrosol
    DIY Witch Hazel Hydrosol, **142**, 143
    Relaxing Lavender Toner and Face Spritz, **20**, 21